Practical Guide to
INTRAUTERINE INSEMINATION (IUI)

Practical Guide to INTRAUTERINE INSEMINATION (IUI)

SECOND EDITION

Chaitanya Nagori
MD (Obstetrics and Gynecology) DGO
Director
Dr Nagori's Institute for Infertility and IVF
Ahmedabad, Gujarat, India

Sonal Panchal
MBBS MD (Radiodiagnosis) PhD
Consultant Sonography Specialist
Dr Nagori's Institute for Infertility and IVF
Ahmedabad, Gujarat, India

JAYPEE

JAYPEE BROTHERS MEDICAL PUBLISHERS
The Health Sciences Publisher
New Delhi | London

Jaypee Brothers Medical Publishers (P) Ltd

Headquarters

Jaypee Brothers Medical Publishers (P) Ltd
EMCA House, 23/23-B
Ansari Road, Daryaganj
New Delhi 110 002, India
Landline: +91-11-23272143, +91-11-23272703
+91-11-23282021, +91-11-23245672
Email: jaypee@jaypeebrothers.com

Corporate Office

Jaypee Brothers Medical Publishers (P) Ltd
4838/24, Ansari Road, Daryaganj
New Delhi 110 002, India
Phone: +91-11-43574357
Fax: +91-11-43574314
Email: jaypee@jaypeebrothers.com

Overseas Office

JP Medical Ltd
83 Victoria Street, London
SW1H 0HW (UK)
Phone: +44 20 3170 8910
Fax: +44 (0)20 3008 6180
Email: info@jpmedpub.com

Website: www.jaypeebrothers.com
Website: www.jaypeedigital.com

Inquiries for bulk sales may be solicited at: jaypee@jaypeebrothers.com

Practical Guide to Intrauterine Insemination (IUI)

First Edition: 2021

Second Edition: **2025**

ISBN: 978-93-6616-653-7

Printed in India at Sterling Graphics Pvt. Ltd.

Dedicated to

My Patients

and

My Students

Preface to the Second Edition

We are very pleased to present the second edition of this book *Practical Guide to Intrauterine Insemination (IUI)*. This book has proved itself up to our expectations for precision of information, to the point, knowledge-based practical tips and as a ready reckoner. It has surely helped several fertility specialists to improve results of intrauterine insemination, which is truly a credit in this era of in vitro fertilization and has proved to be a boon to the patients too residing in remote areas and unable to afford sophisticated ART.

Chaitanya Nagori
Sonal Panchal

Preface to the First Edition

Intrauterine insemination (IUI) is a simple, affordable, and yet effective way of treating infertility. Unfortunately, with the invention and fast innovations in in-vitro fertilization, intrauterine insemination is grossly ignored and also wrongly blamed for poor results. Like any treatment in medicine, the success of IUI also depends on perfection at every step of the procedure, starting from indications or selection of the patient, method, drugs used and even post-procedure care and therapy. In this book, we have tried to give precise and practical tips for every step and every aspect of intrauterine insemination on the basis of our really high intrauterine insemination conception rate and huge number of intrauterine insemination conceptions. We hope that this book will be a ready reckoner for the gynecologists practicing infertility and intrauterine insemination.

Chaitanya Nagori
Sonal Panchal

Acknowledgments

We sincerely acknowledge the entire team of M/s Jaypee Brothers Medical Publishers (P) Ltd, New Delhi, India, especially Shri Jitendar P Vij (Group Chairman) and Mr Ankit Vij (Managing Director), for their support for the publication of the Second Edition of *Practical Guide to Intrauterine Insemination (IUI)*. Our special thanks to Ms Chetna Malhotra (Senior Director—Professional Publishing, Marketing, and Business Development), Ms Pragati Singh (Development Editor) and the entire team, for supporting us during the preparation process of this book.

Contents

CHAPTER 1

Counseling for Intrauterine Insemination

INTRODUCTION

Counseling is the backbone of infertility management. The correct explanation about reproduction and dialogue with the patients help them to conceive. Insler has mentioned in his book that "many patients conceive when they are sitting outside the consulting room". This means that there should be literature placed in the waiting room, handouts given to patients, and there should be elaborative explanatory displays placed in the waiting room that patients can read and would help them clear a lot of their misconceptions about reproduction, which they might be reluctant to clear in person.

In the busy outpatient department (OPD), it is very difficult for a practicing gynecologist to spend time with the patients for counseling. *I shall put forward a few suggestions from my side*:

- There should be good posters placed in the waiting room explaining the physiology of conception.
- Attractive and interesting literature regarding reproductive physiology, causes of infertility, and outline of management should be placed in the waiting room, which should be easily accessible to them.
- We have prepared a small booklet regarding the same in local language, national language, and in English **(Figs. 1A and B)**,

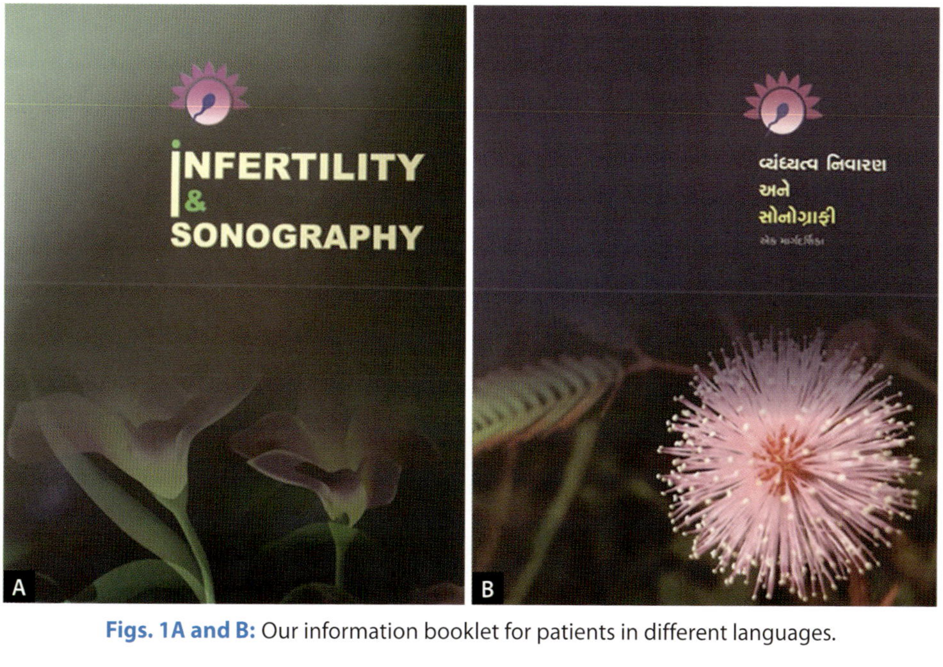

Figs. 1A and B: Our information booklet for patients in different languages.

and is given to every patient once I have done a detailed consultation about their problems with them. This booklet helps the patient to read and understand the things that are discussed once again and take a correct decision about the management of their problem.

Such explanation or literature allows the patient to know what would be the management strategy for their problem and how are we going to deal with their problem and, therefore, they gain confidence and appreciate the treatment that is given.

Moreover, it also would be a great means of propagating the correct knowledge through patients, as they would discuss whatever they have read and understood by reading the book, with their friends. This is very important as if the correct information is not spread in the society, only misconceptions and myths prevail.

One very important suggestion that I would like to give to very busy practitioners—please allot a specific, separate time slot for patients with fertility problems, so that you can patiently listen to them and discuss about the solutions or treatment strategy with them. Remember that the initial counseling and the time spent with the couple play a very vital role in management of the patient.

Now let us elaborate as to how I discuss about various aspects of causes, counseling, and management of infertility.

As infertility is a social stigma in our culture, not only the couple (I mean the husband also) but concerned relatives should also be involved in counseling, so that they would allow the couple to take the correct treatment. The refusal of treatment in majority of cases is by in-laws or parents. Therefore, it is very vital that all the people concerned and all those who are going to play a role in decision making as to whether to continue the treatment or not, should have correct information about infertility. Their myths should be washed out with proper explanation. Explanation should be done in local language, simple for a layman to understand. Eye-to-eye contact is very essential.

When to start the treatment?

85% of the couples conceive within the 1 year of unprotected intercourse and 95% in 2 years. Therefore, if a couple comes earlier than a year and a half of continuous unprotected intercourse (active married life), which is very common at district level and in lower socioeconomic class of people, explaining the above-said fact will increase their faith in you and your treatment.

No invasive investigations such as laparoscopy should be done within these 2 years and nature should be given enough time to work for the couple to achieve pregnancy.

Among noninvasive investigations, semen analysis and midcycle/preovulatory scan are the two investigations that must be done. These will more or less prove the normalcy of the couple and then counseling only can help them conceive.

We have observed that such couples do conceive very often after the treatment is stopped. This is because the stress of treatment is relieved and the patient is relaxed. Moreover, when we are treating these couples, we become too enthusiastic doing some invasive investigation in every cycle one after the other such as Rubin's test (RT), hysterosalpingography (HSG), dilatation and curettage (D and C), laparoscopy, etc. Therefore, when this patient is exhausted and abandons treatment, she conceives spontaneously.

Therefore, remember that counseling is more important than overenthusiastic invasive investigations.

COUNSELING FOR SEMEN ANALYSIS

In 40–50% of couples presenting with fertility problems, male factor is responsible either partially or completely. In our social setup even today, males do not accept this fact and, therefore, they do not agree for examination or investigations. This problem is more prevalent in people who are less educated. Proper counseling is a must with the male partner before subjecting the female partner for treatment for infertility.

The couple must be explained that according to the recent World Health Organization (WHO) criteria 2010, 15 million sperms/mL, 30% motility, and 4% sperms with normal morphology are considered as normal physiological semen criteria. In spite of this even today, we read several laboratories quoting 40–60 million count as normal in their reports. Because of this wrong information and ignorance of laboratory officials and clinicians, several patients take medicines for long periods to increase their sperm count. Remember, when sperm count is 15 million/mL or more, no treatment is required. Up to 86% abnormal sperms is normal and physiological and even patient with 4–14% normal sperms can conceive either naturally or by intrauterine insemination (IUI). Only when <4% of sperms are normal, in vitro fertilization (IVF)/intracytoplasmic sperm injection (ICSI) may be required.

When the sperm count is <15 million/mL, semen analysis must be done at least three times—2 weeks apart and 2 months apart to confirm the diagnosis. These patients should directly not be subjected to IVF or ICSI. Instead, we must try medical treatment for these males to improve the sperm count, so that they can conceive naturally or with IUI. The whole moto of medical management of a subfertile male is not to increase the sperm count 5–10 times or to achieve excellent semen parameters. The moto is to increase the count by a few million so that ICSI can be converted to IVF, IVF to IUI, and perhaps IUI into natural conception. Medical management has been discussed in the Chapter on male infertility.

COUNSELING FOR CERVICAL FACTOR

The cervical factor of infertility is rare at present, as surgeries are not often done on cervix. Frequent D and Cs may damage endocervical glands and epithelium. Cauterization of cervix should be discouraged.

I believe that even today, postcoital test (PCT) is very useful in infertility management. When more than seven sperms are seen per high power field of microscope, 10–12 hours after intercourse, it is an excellent PCT according to WHO standards.

Majority of assisted reproductive technology (ART) textbooks opine that PCT has no significance. I have found it very useful for counseling of the husband. Husband feels that he is normal when PCT is normal. He does not feel guilty and cooperates with his wife for all infertility treatment. So, it may not have a role in patients undergoing ART, but it has a place for IUI and more conservative infertility treatment. Many a times when the couple changes the gynecologist, semen analysis is asked for. If patient has a few reports done earlier, I will rely on PCT. The satisfaction is of highest level for the couple when they see moving sperms under the microscope after 10–12 hours of intercourse.

What information we get from a normal PCT?

- Preovulatory cervical mucus is normal.
- Sperm count is normal.

Moreover, when the patient is shown these moving sperms under microscope even after 12 hours of intercourse, it gives them confidence that both the partners are normal and that helps them conceive.

Patient is explained that these sperms may remain alive for 48–72 hours in most of the patients, and in few, they have also been seen after 7 days. There is a misconception in majority of the couples that intercourse must be done when ovulation occurs. Showing PCT to patients removes this misconception. Cervix acts as a reservoir for sperms, so after the sexual relation even if ovulation occurs in 2–3 days, conception can occur. We can therefore explain the patient that if for conception the intercourse was needed exactly when ovulation occurs, raped girls would not conceive easily. Couple should therefore be advised intercourse at least once in 2–3 days during 10–20 days of 28–30 days cycle. The couple should be clearly told that abstinence of >3 days is not advisable during this period, in natural cycle as well as in stimulated cycles for IUI.

The fertile window of menstrual cycle precedes the day of ovulation by 5–6 days and likelihood of pregnancy is highest when intercourse occurs 2 days before ovulation. Intercourse on the day of ovulation is less effective and success rate is almost zero on the day after ovulation.[1,2] Coital frequency of twice or thrice a week during fertile period is equally effective. But once a week reduces the chance of pregnancy by 40%.

Majority of the couples believe that if IUI is done, it is better to have abstinence before to get good sperm count. But this is not true. An abstinence of >3–4 days does not increase the count, instead the percentage of dead sperms in this semen increases. Therefore, intercourse should not be planned; it should be absolutely voluntary and can be done irrespective of the day of IUI.

Abstinence is one of the causes for failed IUI. Let me explain, why and how!! In majority of gynecology clinics, where there is no IVF setup, the semen preparation laboratory is not adequately equipped, and so the semen preparation is suboptimal and so chances of conception are less. Moreover, patient keeps abstinence before IUI, so the chance of natural conception also is denied. As a result, patient does not conceive when she is on treatment but conceives spontaneously when she abandons treatment. Remember, therefore, intercourse at regular intervals in the fertile period is absolutely essential.

Majority of couples with long-term infertility have lost the charm of their marital relations. Their intercourses are only planned and compulsory, only targeted for childbearing. They must be explained that child is only a byproduct. Main thing is the love and affection, intercourse is just an expression of this feeling and results in conception. Counseling can help them to regain the charm of their marriage. All myths regarding intercourse must be discussed and sorted out, e.g., posture, position, timing, washing, etc.

COUNSELING FOR UTERINE FACTOR

This is to be discussed with the patient after a 3D ultrasound, as this is a gold standard for congenital uterine malformations and endometrial pathologies. Patient also can see and understand these 3D pictures and the optimum management then can be easily explained. Fibroids <4–5 cm in size and not touching the endometrium do not require removal. Patient can also be convinced explaining them how the embryo traverses from the tube to the uterus and implants in the endometrium.

Majority of the patients have a wrong concept that D and C helps conception. This is a myth and should be clarified. D and C should not be done in modern infertility practice. The only role today of D and C is to exclude endometrial tuberculosis (TB) by either histopathology or TB polymerase chain reaction (PCR) of the endometrial sample along with culture. D and C must not be done to diagnose luteal phase defect or to check whether the endometrium is in proliferative phase or secretory phase.

COUNSELING FOR TUBAL FACTOR

Patient must be explained that fertilization occurs in fallopian tube and after 4–5 days, embryo comes to settle in the uterus.

This explanation is also useful to counsel, if the patient gets an ectopic pregnancy. Tubal evaluation is very important in infertility practice. RT should not be done. Laparoscopy is the gold standard for evaluation of the tubes and tubo-ovarian relationship.

Patient should be explained that at the time of ovulation, fimbrial end of the tube covers the ovary, a negative pressure of 1 mm of Hg is created due to movements of the cilia, this sucks the ovum from the follicle, into the tubal lumen **(Fig. 2)**. So, ovum does not separate and release from the follicle to roll into the tubal lumen, but tube is vital and instrumental to suck the ovum into tubal lumen. Therefore, it is important that tubo-ovarian relation should be healthy, a patent tube is not sufficient. HSG gives us only incomplete information about the patency of the tube. This can be replaced by sonosalpingography (SSG). This explains the patient that in spite of patent tubes on other tests, why is laparoscopy required.

Now, microsurgery is almost replaced by ART for pathological tubes. Results of microsurgery are very good in tubo-tubal anastomosis in patients with tubal ligation (TL) especially laparoscopic tubal ligation. Therefore, in young patients where TL is done, and patient then again wishes a pregnancy, microsurgery should be offered as an alternative to ART, as it is a one-time procedure and patient gets a breathing time for up to 2 years.

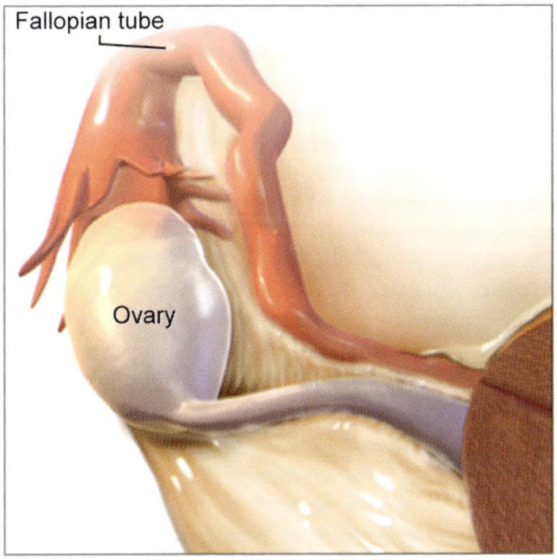

Fig. 2: Diagrammatic demonstration of tubo-ovarian relation.

COUNSELING FOR OVARIAN CAUSES

Patient should be counseled that ovum is released from the ovary only once in a month and it survives for 6–8 hours. Sperms that are stored in the cervix can stay live for at least 48 hours to up to maximum 7 days, and these can reach the ova and conception can occur. Though patient should also be explained that the chances of conception are maximum, if the sperms are available for the ovum soon after ovulation. That would also explain them the importance of the time of IUI. Ovulation can be confirmed by serum progesterone levels assessed on Day 21–22. Daily sonography is not required just to confirm whether the ovulation has occurred or not, if no intervention such as IUI or ovulation trigger for timed intercourse is planned. Basal body temperature record and cervical mucus do not help much in deciding the time of ovulation and mode of management.

UNEXPLAINED INFERTILITY

About 5–10% of patients are infertile in spite of everything being normal. They have normal semen analysis, normal endoscopy, normal luteal phase, and normal endocrinological reports. These are the ideal patients for IUI. Six cycles of superovulation with IUI must be tried before subjecting the patient for ART when the patient's age is <35 years. IUI is the choice of treatment for idiopathic/unexplained infertility rather than IVF.

The rationale for IUI is increasing the number of available motile sperms to reach the ovum, which is morphologically normal for fertilization.

Intrauterine insemination is unfortunately the least standardized management of infertility. IUI is blamed for low pregnancy rate. But, meticulous selection of patient, stimulation protocol, ultrasound monitoring, and good semen preparation combined with IUI give excellent pregnancy rate. It bypasses vaginal acidity and cervical hostility. But, simultaneously accurate timing of IUI is necessary as reservoir function of cervical crypts is escaped and sperm has to travel only a short distance to approach ovum.

"Treatment independent pregnancy among infertile couple" is a landmark paper for patients who have patent tubes and fair sperm quality.[3]

To maximize the health outcome of population with minimum possible use of resources, cost-effectiveness of intervention is an important consideration in any healthcare system. Infertility treatment in our country is not covered either by government or by insurance companies. So, the choice of treatment is driven by financial consideration rather than best effectiveness. Success rate should be considered by spending same amount of money rather than number of cycles. For example, the cost of one IVF is almost same, as it would cost for 4–6 cycles of IUI. Considering a patient of unexplained infertility, male subfertility, or dysovulatory infertility, pregnancy rate of 4–6 cycles will be much higher than one cycle of IVF. So, if proper counseling is done, patient will first opt for IUI.

Even the practice committee of American Society for Reproductive Medicine (ASRM), 2012 recommends starting with less invasive treatment such as IUI and move to more aggressive intervention such as IVF, if IUI is unsuccessful or when patient is elderly, or it is long-term infertility.[4]

Counseling is to be for the whole procedure of IUI. Most of the patients come with previous IUI failures in many cycles. They believe that IUI, just the procedure, gives them pregnancy. It should be emphasized that each and every step of IUI is very important. If all steps are not performed properly, IUI does not give the results. For example, following steps should be discussed:

- Stimulation protocol with gonadotropins
- US monitoring by at least color Doppler
- Proper timing of IUI and its method
- Luteal support
- Semen preparation

All the steps combined together if done systematically, then and then, IUI can give good pregnancy rates.

I have discussed "counseling for IUI" in detail specifically because patients have wrong concepts and even consultants refer for IVF after few IUI failures, which are not done optimally.

Whenever patient is under treatment, she can do all her regular activities such as household work, exercise, office work, etc. All these activities do not decrease the pregnancy rate. On the contrary, they have the beneficial role for the patient.

COUNSELING FOR DONOR INSEMINATION

Counseling for donor insemination should be done to all the patients who have very low count or azoospermia before proceeding to ICSI. Many patients who cannot afford ART may opt for AID.

Donor should be unknown and all the norms and standard operating procedures of Indian Council of Medical Research (ICMR) for donor semen should be followed strictly. Sample should be ordered from registered semen bank. Many a times, couple ask for relative as their donor, which should be strongly discouraged. Donor and couple should never know each other and these details should be kept confidential. Child in future can ask about the genetic prints after 18 years, but that information also should be given without personal identification of the donor.

COUNSELING FOR IN VITRO FERTILIZATION

There are lots of misconceptions prevailing for IVF treatment regarding three aspects:

1. Indications
2. Results
3. Cost

Indications

It must be clearly understood that IVF is the first choice in only those patients who have bilateral tubal block, severe endometriosis, or severe male factor infertility. IVF may be done in patients with unexplained infertility only when six well-tried superovulations with IUI cycles have failed to give pregnancy. Dysovulatory infertility such as polycystic ovary syndrome (PCOS) is not an indication of IVF.

Results

Patients believe that IVF is like a fast food and a sure shot solution to infertility. They have been misled about the same. They must be explained that the results of IVF in the best centers of the world are:

- 30% in first cycle
- 40–45% in second cycle
- 50–55% in three cycles
- 60–65% in four cycles
- 65–70% in five cycles
- 70–73% in six cycles

Therefore, patients who do not have absolute indications for IVF should be given a chance of IUI instead of taking them for IVF because about six superovulations with IUI cycles cost the same as one IVF cycle, with more chances of success.

Cost

In vitro fertilization is a very expensive procedure. Its cost includes charges for gonadotropins and medicines, which comprises the largest amount, nearing ₹ 60,000–80,000 depending on the consumption by the patient. The second highest cost is of disposables and media. This is also about ₹ 10,000–15,000. Over and above this, the cost also includes that of the IVF consultant, embryologist, anesthetist, etc. Therefore, it must be understood when we try to cut-off the cost, one has to compromise on drug quality and disposables. This would definitely compromise with the results also. Many a times when packages are fixed, compromise occurs in treatment.

CARRY HOME MESSAGE

- Counseling plays very important role in infertility management.
- 15 million counts with 30% motility with 4% normal sperms are new WHO, 2010 criteria.
- Seven motile sperms/high-power field (hpf) are excellent PCT.
- D and C is done only to rule out tuberculosis.
- Laparoscopy is gold standard for tubal evaluation.
- Serum progesterone on Day 21 indicates ovulation.
- Six cycles of IUI should be tried in unexplained infertility before ART.
- When taking patients for ART, results and cost must be discussed with the patient.

REFERENCES

1. Stanford JB, Dunson DB. Effects of sexual intercourse patterns in time to pregnancy studies. Am J Epidemiol. 2007;165(9):1088-95.
2. Practice Committee of American Society for Reproductive Medicine in collaboration with Society for Reproductive Endocrinology and Infertility. Optimizing natural fertility. Fertil Steril. 2008;90(5 Suppl):S1-6.
3. Collins JA, Wrixon W, Janes LB, Wilson EH. Treatment-independent pregnancy among infertile couples. N Engl J Med. 1983;309(20):1201-6.
4. Van den Boofard NM, Bensdorp AJ, Rengerink KO, Barnhart K, Bhattacharya S, Custers IM, et al. Prognostic profiles and the effectiveness of assisted conception: secondary analyses of individual patient data. Hum Reprod Update. 2014;20(1):141-51.

CHAPTER 2

Diagnostic Work-up Before Intrauterine Insemination

INTRODUCTION

Work-up of both the partners is required but should be restricted to the tests that contribute to the prediction of effectiveness of intrauterine insemination (IUI).

HISTORY TAKING

Try to get detailed history about any medicines that patient is taking or surgery done for both the partners. History of chewing tobacco, smoking, alcohol, or hard drugs is important, as it may contribute to infertility. Lifestyle details must also be asked for. It often happens that work timings or burden of one/both the partners may be the cause of infertility.

This history is very important, including the history of previous infertility treatment taken, also including IUIs done. This will decide how many IUIs can be further done. If no gonadotropin IUI cycles are done or the cycles are not monitored by color Doppler for assessment of follicular quality and endometrial receptivity, I will not consider these IUIs adequate.

LOCAL AND GENERAL EXAMINATION

For female partner, routine per abdominal, per vaginal, and per speculum examination of the patient is required to find out any evident abnormalities in abdomen that may be associated with or may be causative of infertility. Though prevaginal examination can be avoided, if the transvaginal ultrasound is done by the gynecologist himself. Local examination of the male partner consists of per abdominal examination and examination of the scrotum, if required, in standing position and with Valsalva to assess for varicocele.

General examination of both the partners includes assessment of vital parameters such as heart rate, blood pressure, respiratory rate, etc. Patient's height and weight are also noted along with calculated body mass index (BMI).

A BMI between 25–29.9 kg/m^2 or >30 kg/m^2 does not appear to have a negative effect on live birth rate after IUI. Obesity may be associated with higher risk of biochemical pregnancy after IUI.[1]

DETAILED ULTRASOUND SCAN

It is done to assess uterus, ovaries, and tubes for any pathologies and their impact on fertility potential of the patient. This scan ideally should be done between day 6 and 7 till day 18 of a normal length cycle. The endometrium is multi-layered during this period and, therefore, Müllerian duct abnormalities and endometrial pathologies can be diagnosed more confidently **(Figs. 1A and B)**. One may also look for fibroids **(Fig. 2A)**, adenomyosis, or other uterine pathologies and also for ovarian and adnexal lesions such as endometriomas or hydrosalpinges **(Figs. 2B and C)**. But this may be considered a pilot scan and may be done when patient presents for the first time.

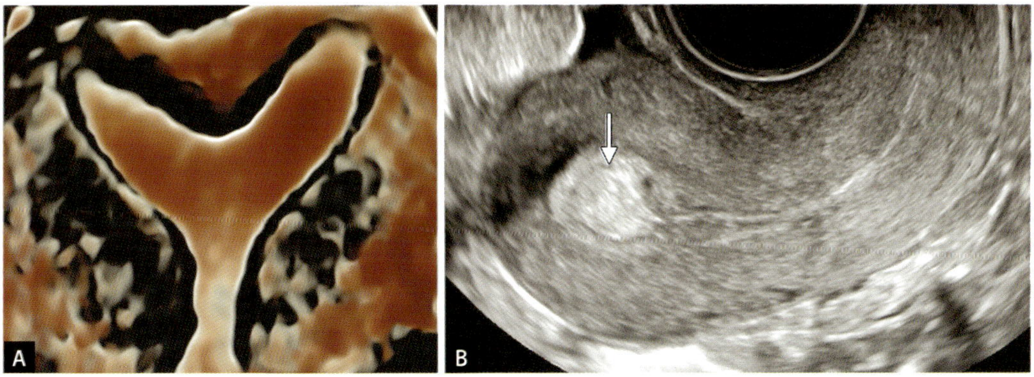

Figs. 1A and B: (A) 3D ultrasound showing subseptate uterus; (B) B-mode ultrasound showing endometrial polyp (arrow).

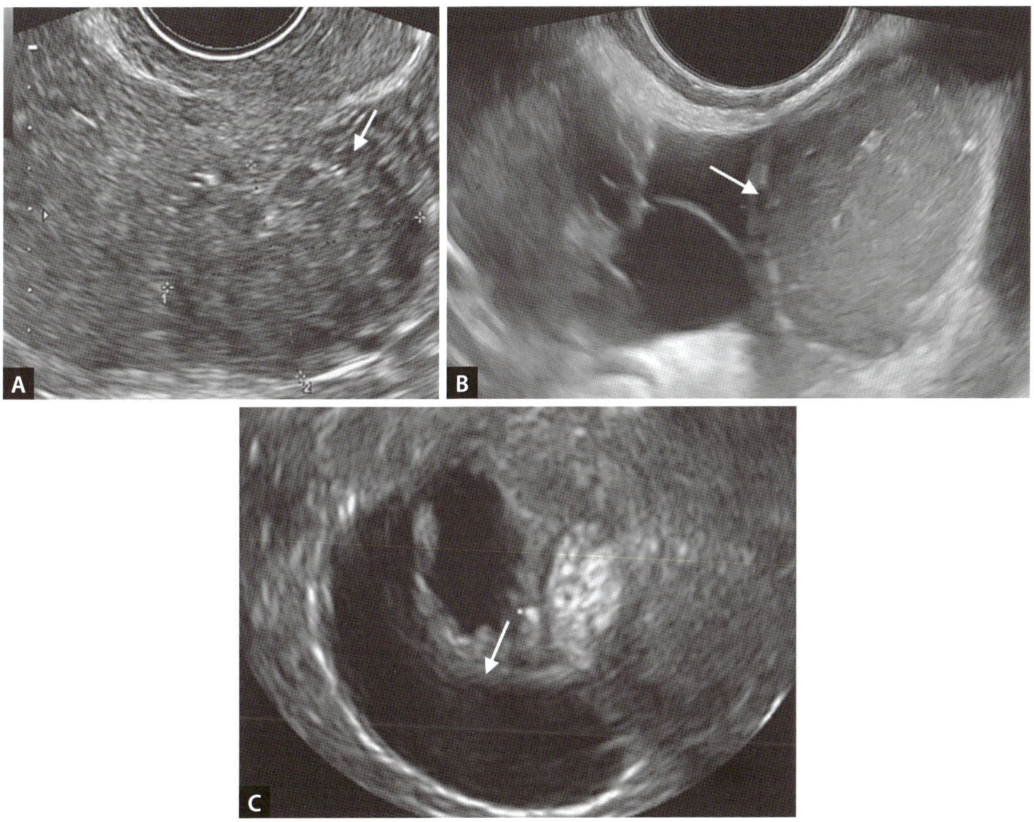

Figs. 2A to C: (A) B-mode ultrasound showing fibroid in uterus (arrow); (B) B-mode ultrasound showing endometrioma (arrow); (C) B-mode ultrasound of hydrosalpinx (arrow).

BASELINE ULTRASOUND SCAN AND PREOVULATORY SCAN

This has been discussed in detail in the chapter on ultrasound monitoring. Baseline scan is essential to know the ovarian reserve and response. This will help to decide the stimulation protocol and the dose of gonadotropin required. It also will help to diagnose polycystic ovaries (PCO) **(Fig. 3)** and modify the treatment accordingly.

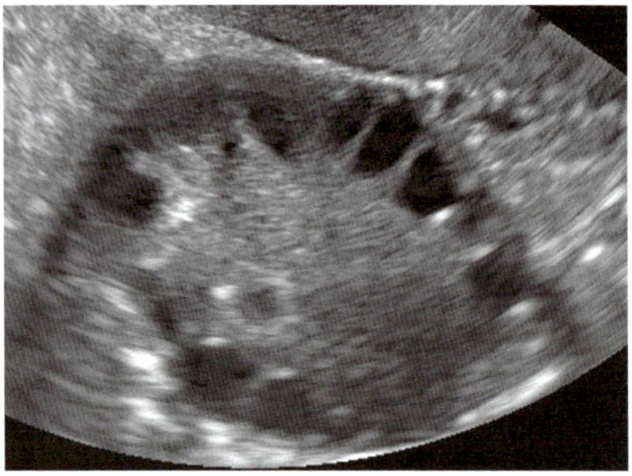

Fig. 3: B-mode ultrasound of polycystic ovary.

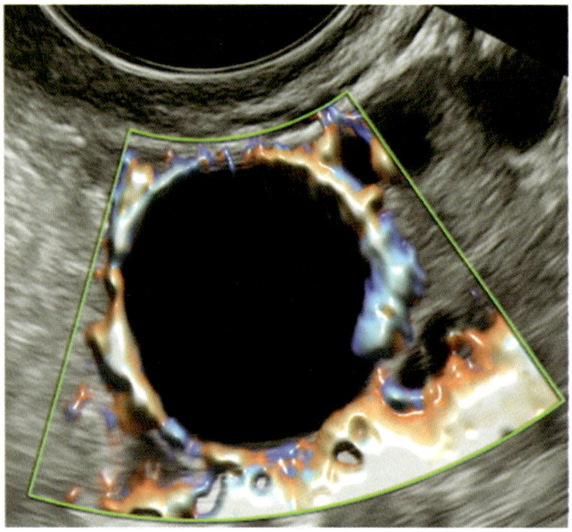

Fig. 4: Color Doppler of mature follicle.

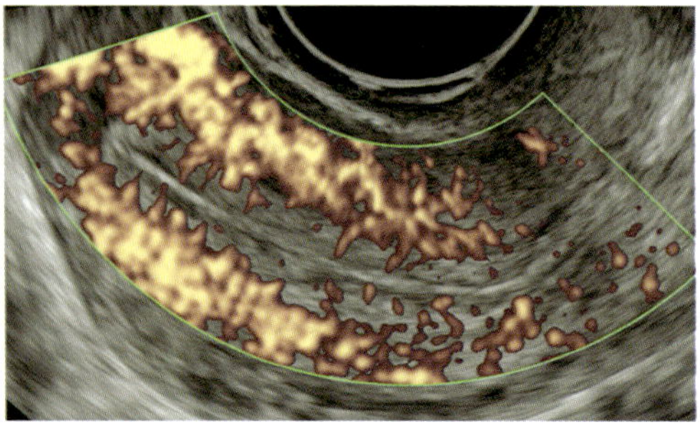

Fig. 5: Power Doppler of receptive endometrium.

Preovulatory scan is done with color Doppler to assess the follicular quality and maturity and endometrial receptivity **(Figs. 4 and 5)**. This is an important guide to decide the stimulation protocol and to add adjuvants to ovulation induction.

ROUTINE LABORATORY INVESTIGATIONS

These include complete blood count, prothrombin time (PT), surface antigen of the hepatitis B (HbsAg), HIV, SGPT, and serum creatinine. Urine routine and microscopy test is to be done. Hormonal investigations required would be serum thyroid-stimulating hormone (TSH) and serum prolactin. Though most practitioners get an infertility package done, it is very important to understand that estrogen, progesterone, follicle-stimulating hormone (FSH), luteinizing hormone (LH), and androgen, all done on the same day, do not have a clinical relevance. These tests may be suggested very selectively, as most practical information about these hormones can be judged by ultrasound and Doppler, which is otherwise also done for monitoring. Insulin resistance test is to be done to confirm or exclude polycystic ovarian syndrome (PCOS) and also to decide the line of treatment.

Insulin resistance is calculated as fasting glucose/insulin, if <4.5, it indicates insulin resistance or 2-hour glucose tolerance and 2-hour insulin response test can be done **(Tables 1 and 2)**.

Any other specific laboratory investigation that may be suggested and dependent on the history may be done.

TABLE 1: Values of glucose on 2-hour glucose tolerance test.

2-hour glucose tolerance test (after 75 g of glucose):
- *Normal:* <140 mg/dL
- *Impaired:* 140–190 mg/dL
- *Noninsulin-dependent diabetes mellitus:* >200 mg/dL

TABLE 2: Insulin levels on 2-hour insulin response test.

2-hour insulin response (after 75 g of glucose):
- *Insulin resistance very likely:* 100–150 μU/mL
- *Insulin resistance:* 151–300 μU/mL
- *Severe insulin resistance:* >300 μU/mL

TABLE 3: Normal semen analysis parameters according to World Health Organization (WHO), 2010 guidelines.[2]

Seminal parameters	*Lower reference value*
Volume	1.5 mL
pH	7.2
Concentration	15 million/mL
Total number of sperms	39 million/ejaculate
Motility	40% total 32% progressive
Vitality	58% sperms alive/ ejaculate
Morphology	4% normal shape

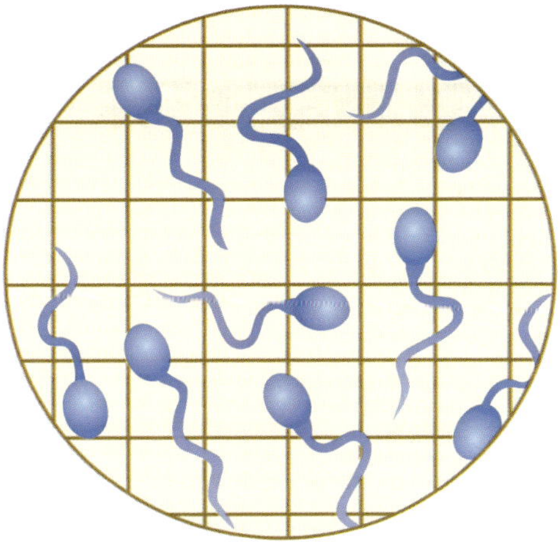

Fig. 6: Diagrammatic presentation of normal postcoital test (PCT) as seen under the microscope.

SEMEN ANALYSIS

It should be done in detail, as this will help to decide which semen wash method should be used for a particular patient and what modifications will be required **(Table 3)**.

These are the normal parameters for a semen sample, but these are not predictors of pregnancy after IUI.[3,4] Total motile sperm count (TMSC) gives a better idea about the same. TMSC is calculated as (volume of the semen sample × concentration of sperms 10^6/mL) × progressive motility.

According to the Dutch gynecological and general practitioner guidelines:[3]

- Mild male subfertility, if TMSC is >3 × 10^6, can conceive with IUI.
- Moderate male subfertility, if TMSC is 1–3 × 10^6, requires IVF.
- Severe male subfertility, if TMSC is <1 × 10^6, requires ICSI
- Post-wash sperm count of 0.8 × 10^6 - 5 × 10^6 TMSC is accepted.[4]

Antisperm antibodies (ASAs) can be tested, if sperm agglutination is found, but its role is doubtful.

POSTCOITAL TEST

In cervical factor, infertility or abnormal postcoital test (PCT) showed no benefit of IUI over 6 months of no treatment.[5] But, it has great psychological impact on the couple when the test is positive, and patient can see the motile sperms on under the microscope **(Fig. 6)**. We routinely do PCT after 10–12 hours of intercourse in preovulatory period. According to WHO criteria, excellent PCT correlates with high pregnancy rate.

Postcoital test parameters according to WHO, 1976:

- *Normal:* (A)—Seven sperms without agglutination
- *Inconclusive:* (B)—One to seven sperms, no agglutination, and good progressive movement
- *Suspected immunological:* (C)—Agglutination regardless of number of sperms per HPF
- *Abnormal:* (D)—Nonmoving sperms only
- *Abnormal:* (E)—No sperms

TUBAL FACTOR

Rubin's test should never be done for assessment of tubal patency, as it is not reliable. For tubal factor, hysterolaparoscopy is a must, which can assess tubo-ovarian relations. It has already been discussed in the chapter on "Indications for IUI", how ovulation occurs. So, only laparoscopy can establish tubo-ovarian relation status. I have not done any hysterosalpingography (HSG) since last 20 years for tubal assessment, as it gives incomplete information with low accuracy, and it is a very painful procedure. Blocked tubes in HSG may turn out to be normal and it may further cause infection. If preovulatory scan is done and uterus and ovaries are freely mobile and there is no pathology in the tube, then 3–4 IUIs should be done before laparoscopy. No tubal patency test is done before 30 years of age unless indicated or suspected due to relevant history that may suggest possibility of tubal damage. Tubal pathology, if leads to hydrosalpinx, will be seen on ultrasound or tubal block may be indicated by adhesions. In these cases, laparoscopy is a must. In present era of advanced ultrasound technology, endoscopy should be only therapeutic-operative and not diagnostic. If there is a doubt in fimbrial end status, 3D hysterosalpingocontrast sonography (HyCoSy) can well demonstrate the pathology **(Fig. 7)**.

Saline Infusion Salpingography Technique

Saline infusion salpingography (SSG) is done in mid-proliferative phase (Days 6–10 of a typical 28-day cycle), after menstruation stops but before ovulation occurs, to reduce the risk of disturbing an early pregnancy. Oral analgesic, ibuprofen 400–600 mg may be given 1–2 hours before the procedure. Preprocedural screenings for infections like chlamydia and/or prophylactic oral antibiotics are recommended. Strict asepsis is essential. A detailed transvaginal ultrasound scan is done to assess the position of pelvic organs and to rule out any pathologies, which would come in the way of the procedure. Moreover, any free fluid in pelvis is also checked for.

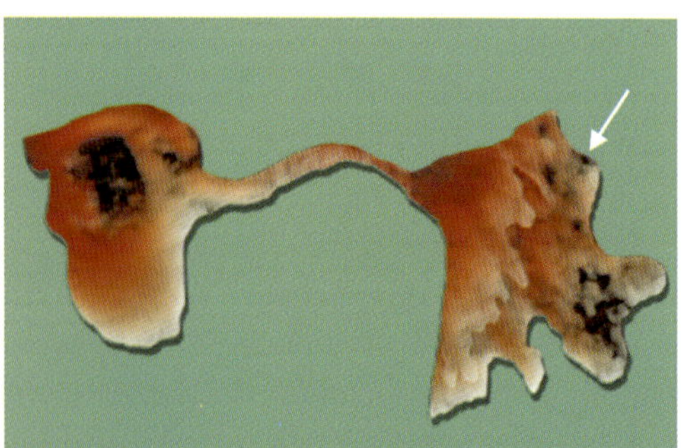

Fig. 7: 3D hysterosalpingocontrast sonography (HyCoSy) image showing a patent unilateral tube with fimbrial end (arrow).

After finishing the primary pre-procedure scan, speculum is placed in the vagina to visualize the cervix. Vagina and cervix are cleaned with antiseptic solution. Cervix is fixed with tenaculum to align it with uterus. An 8F balloon catheter or a cannula, especially devised for saline infusion sonography or hysterosalpingography, is attached to a 10-mL syringe prefilled with saline. The catheter is introduced through cervix into the uterus. Balloon is distended with 1–2 mL of distilled water or normal saline and is placed just beyond the internal os. Alternatives to this, catheter are pediatric feeding tubes or small gage Foley catheter. Once the catheter is fixed, tenaculum and speculum are removed and transvaginal probe is introduced into the vagina for further assessment.

Saline is injected through the catheter slowly. Scanning is done to assess the uterine cavity that is distended by saline and also passage of saline (fluid) seen through the tubes. Spill of saline from fimbrial end is seen as fluid flow surrounding the ovary and its collection in pelvis on B-mode scanning. Absence of spill may indicate blockage. It is not always possible to document the spill from the fimbrial end of individual tube. In such cases, fluid accumulation in pouch of Douglas confirms patency of at least one fallopian tube. In patients with bilateral block, distension of the uterine cavity causes severe pain and no spill is observed.

Adding color Doppler may increase the efficiency and accuracy of SIS for assessment of tubal patency. Large color box is used to cover the entire ovary but not to overlap the myometrium, show saline injection will lead to color blush in the color box, indicating a patent tube and no blush confirms block tube. During injection of saline, patient's movement must be strictly restricted to avoid color artefacts.

HyCoSy (Hysterocontrast Salpingography) Technique

The technique for HyCoSy is the same as for saline infusion salpingography. As delineation of the tube is better with HyCoSy, total amount of contrast needed is as less as 2–3 mL per tube. For diagnosis of tubal patency, two to three observation phases per tube are needed, with an observation period of continuous flow of about 10 s. Visualization of long segments of tube beyond intramural part of the tube usually indicates patency, though whole tube must be observed, and spill should be confirmed. Appearance or increase in the fluid in pouch of Douglas may be an indirect sign of tubal patency, the same as for SIS. HyCoSy has several advantages over saline infusion salpingography, like it helps clearer visualization of uterine cavity, better assessment of tubal lumen and fimbriae, clearer visualization of spill, and a more exact localization of site of block. Having defined the contrast filling in the tubes, 3D is switched on and volumes are acquired for each side independently.

Rendering is done in front-back viewing direction. Surface-enhanced mode is used. Threshold is set to make the contrast path more obvious. MagiCut (electronic scalpel) is then used to cut all shadows other than the contrast path. Then HD-live rendering mode is switched on and direction of the light is adjusted to visualize the fimbriae and spill to its best.

Chlamydial antibody test (CAT) is useful to find outpatients with high risk of tubal pathology. Direct questions may be asked to inquire for tubal pathology, in cases where there is a possibility that patient may have missed the specific history or has hidden it for a purpose.

ROUTINE OVARIAN RESERVE TESTS

These are not required before IUI. Baseline ultrasound with antral follicle count (AFC) gives all the information. In IUI, more ova are not required as in IVF. One or two good follicles, if can be produced by ovulation induction, good results can be achieved, and this is possible even in low ovarian reserve. We always depend on AFC rather than anti-Müllerian hormone (AMH). In majority of patients with AMH between 0.3 and 1, 2–3 follicles will almost always develop every cycle and results of IUI are always good. So even though it is a drastic statement, IUI has a definite role in low AMH with advancing age.

Vagios et al.[6] analyzed outcome of 1861 gonadotropin ovulation induction with IUI cycles in 821 patients. Women with low AMH (<0.75 ng/mL) had lower cumulative pregnancy rates over 3 cycles. Women with AMH <0.4 ng/mL, had twice the risk of abortions. But surprisingly women with low AMH had a significantly higher risk of multiple pregnancies. Doses of gonadotropins and method of AMH estimation, having changed now, women with low AMH are more likely to continue with gonadotropin stimulated IUI cycles, while high AMH patients have more anovulatory cycles and so after a trial of few IUI cycles, these patients may require to go for IVF. The practice committee report recommends oral ovarian stimulation in diminished ovarian reserve.[7]

LUTEAL PHASE SCAN

It is essential to assess corpus luteal function and exclude possibility of luteal phase abnormalities, which may be the cause of infertility.

AGE

Age is the single factor that decreases AFC. Ours being a tertiary center for infertility, majority of the patients come after 8–10 years of infertility and are above 35 years of age. In spite of that, excellent pregnancy rate can be maintained by gonadotropin stimulation and ovulation monitoring with color Doppler even when IUI is done.

OUR DATA

We have 189 IUI pregnancies, in cases with previous 3 or more IVF failures. Majority of these patients were advised ovum donation elsewhere. So, my strong carry home message is "*do not underestimate the strength of IUI*".

According to what is documented in one of the studies, when age of the male partner is >35 years, it may be a factor causative of poor IUI outcome.[8]

I absolutely do not agree with this, as the only factor in male that affects the success of IUI according to my experience is the sperm count. As mentioned earlier, majority of our patients and therefore their male partners are also >35 years of age. This is further discussed in the chapter of factors affecting the success of IUI.

CARRY HOME MESSAGE

- Detailed history including the details of previous IUIs and how were these done.
- Baseline scan is essential to rule out pathologies and decide stimulation protocol.
- Insulin resistance test and stromal volume with 3D ultrasound are important tests for treatment.
- Total motile sperm concentration can give better idea for prognosis.
- Excellent PCT gives positive psychological impact.
- Tubo-ovarian relations can be assessed by laparoscopy only.
- Routine ovarian reserve tests are not required.

REFERENCES

1. Whynott RM, Summers KM, Van Voorhis BJ, Mejia RB. Effect of body mass index on intrauterine insemination cycle success. Fertil Steril. 2021;115(1):221-8).
2. World Health organization. Laboratory Manual for the Examination of Human Semen and Semen-cervical Mucus Interaction, 5th edition. New York: Cambridge University Press; 2010. p. 287.
3. Van Weert JM, Verhoeve H, Mil BW. Diagnostic work up before IUI. In: Cohlen B, Ombelet W (Eds). Intrauterine Insemination: Evidence-based Guidelines for Daily Practice. Boca Raton, London, New York: CRC Press, Taylor and Francis Group; 2014.
4. Van Weert JM, Repping S, Van Voorhis B, Bossuyt P, Van der Veen F, Mil BW. The performance of the postwash total motile sperm count at the time of intrauterine insemination from the prediction of pregnancy: a meta-analysis. Fertil Steril. 2004;82(3):612-20.
5. Steures P, Van der Steeg JW, Hompes PG, Bossuyt PM, Habbema JD, Eijkemans MJ, et al. Effectiveness of intrauterine insemination in subfertile couples with an isolated cervical factor: a randomized clinical trial. Fertil Steril. 2007;88(6):1692-6.
6. Vagios S, Hsu JY, Sacha CR, Dimitriadis I, Christou G, James KF, et al. Pretreatment anti-müllerian hormone levels and outcomes of ovarian stimulation with gonadotropins/intrauterine insemination cycles. Fertil Steril. 2021;116:422-30.
7. Practice Committee of American Society for Reproductive Medicine. Evidence-based treatments for couples with unexplained infertility: a guideline. Fertil Steril. 2020;113:305-22.
8. Henkel R, Maass AG, Schuppe HC, Jung A, Schubert J. Molecular aspects of aging sperm. Fertil Steril. 2005;84(5):1430-7.

CHAPTER 3

Indications of Intrauterine Insemination

INTRODUCTION

Appropriate patient selection is the most important step in determining the success of intrauterine insemination (IUI). IUI should be done for following indications:

- Unexplained infertility
- Ovarian dysfunction
- Male subfertility
- Endometriosis
- Cervical factor
- Immunological factor
- Single tube
- Frozen sample IUI
- Human immunodeficiency virus (HIV) discordant males
- Donor sperms
- Sexual disorders

Let us discuss the role of IUI in individual indication.

UNEXPLAINED INFERTILITY

Incidence of unexplained infertility is 10–15%. In unexplained infertility, superovulation with IUI has higher pregnancy rate than only superovulation.[1] The concept is to get the best ova by ovulation induction with good semen wash to get maximum number of most motile and healthy sperms and put those as close to the ova as possible. Unexplained infertility is the first in the list of indications of IUI. It is not at the top of the list in indications for IVF. Most common indication for IVF, instead, is block tube followed by low sperm count, grade III and IV endometriosis, etc. and then unexplained infertility.

So, do not rush for IVF in patients with unexplained infertility. We have documented a series of 189 patients who have conceived with IUI after three or more IVF cycles failed elsewhere. In this group, majority of the patients had unexplained infertility. Spontaneous pregnancy after IVF failure is also not uncommon in patients with unexplained infertility.

In EXIUI study, expectant management versus IUI in unexplained infertility and poor pregnancy prognosis was studied. It was concluded that IUI with ovarian stimulation is superior over expectant management. Live birth rate with IUI was 33% as compared to only 13% for expectant management.[2]

Compared with 3 cycles of IUI, single cycle of ART was estimated to have similar probability of live birth but slightly higher risk of multiple pregnancy, preterm birth and NICU (neonatal intensive care unit) admission. This study showed 26% pregnancy rate in IVF between the age of 18–40 years and 27% for IUI group. For women aged more than 40 years, IVF had a better pregnancy rate.[3]

In patients with unexplained infertility[4] conception rates after different treatment protocols are mentioned in **Table 1**.

Using recombinant follicle-stimulating hormone (rFSH) instead of HMG may improve the results further, to our opinion. Ovarian stimulation with IUI is more effective in patients even with poor prognosis, rather than IVF, i.e., long-term infertility, elderly patients, and primary infertility.

However, Cochrane review, 2016 did not find conclusive evidence for difference in live birth with timed intercourse with or without stimulation.[5] It has been confirmed that controlled ovarian hyperstimulation and IUI significantly improve IUI results.[1]

OVARIAN DYSFUNCTION

Correction of ovulatory derangement with controlled ovarian hyperstimulation combined with IUI gives better results. This helps to develop more than one follicles and that also helps correct subtle hormonal derangements and helps patient conceive. Absolute pregnancy rate is higher with multiple follicles as compared to monofollicular growth.[6]

MALE SUBFERTILITY

Table 2 indicates a normal semen sample and the males with semen parameters matching to this are considered to have normal fertility potential. When the motile sperm count is <10 million before wash, it is considered male subfertility. Mild ovarian stimulation with IUI in these patients gives very good results.[8] IUI is done when the count is low, poor motility, poor morphology, or other abnormal semen parameters. When sperm count is less and 0.8–5.0 million motile sperms are inseminated, conception hardly occurs.[8] This is a wide range though. Most clinics use a cut-off of 0.8–1.0 million. John Balasch recommends 2 million count and 4% normal morphology post-wash as eligible for IUI. In a couple with infertility but normal male factor, single IUI is enough but for male factor, double IUI, one IUI before ovulation and another at the time of ovulation, gives better conception rates compared with single IUI.[9]

Always try to improve the count by medical line of treatment, so that IVF can be converted into IUI. Unfortunately, research on the drugs that can improve the count has been completely ceased and all the patients are taken for assisted reproductive technology (ART) since IVF came into practice. But in India, neither the Government nor the insurance company pays or compensates for the expenses done for infertility treatment. So, it is very important to keep the expenses to minimum without compromising the

TABLE 1: Conception rates with different treatment protocols in patients with unexplained infertility.

Natural cycle + IUI	3.8%
CC + IUI	8.3%
HMG + IUI	17%
IVF	20%

(CC: clomiphene citrate; HMG: human menopausal gonadotropin; IUI: intrauterine insemination; IVF: in vitro fertilization)

TABLE 2: Difference in the normal semen criteria according to WHO criteria 1999 and 2010.[7]

Parameters	*2010 (5th Edition)*	*2021 (6th Edition)*
Semen volume (mL)	1.5 (1.4 – 1.7)	1.4 (1.3 – 1.5)
Total sperms (10^6 per ejaculate)	≥39 (33 – 46)	≥39 (35 – 40)
Sperm conc (10^6 per mL)	≥15 (12 – 16)	≥16 (15 – 18)
Total motility (%)	≥40 (38 – 42)	≥ 42 (40 – 43)
Progressive motility (%)	≥32 (31 – 34)	≥ 30 (29 – 31)
Non progressive motility (%)	1	1
Immotile sperm (%)	22	20 (19 – 20)
Vitality (%)	≥58 (55 – 63)	≥54 (50 – 56)
Normal forms (%)	≥4 (3 – 4)	≥4 (3.9 – 4.0)

results. Improving the count with drugs is therefore a better option for mild-to-moderate male subfertility, so that the sperm count may improve and the couple may conceive with IUI instead of IVF. Discussion on medical management of male infertility is out of the scope of this book. Antioxidants, varicocele ligation, and antibiotics with anti-inflammatory agents may help to improve sperm count.

ENDOMETRIOSIS

Better results with IUI can be obtained in mild endometriosis [AFS (American Fertility Society) grade 1 and 2]. In these cases, tubo-ovarian relations are not grossly disturbed and so pregnancy rate is very good with IUI. But in stage III and IV endometriosis, tubo-ovarian relations are disturbed and so pregnancy rate is poor with IUI. In these patients, IVF is the only option available.

Mild endometriosis patients are treated as unexplained infertility and they benefit from superovulation with IUI when two to three follicles grow and mature. Up to six cycles of IUI may be offered, as these increase the chances of pregnancy.[10] Ablation of endometriotic lesions rather than diagnostic laparoscopy improves spontaneous pregnancy rates. But, stage III and IV endometriosis gives only 2–3% pregnancy rate and for these patients, ART is recommended.

CERVICAL FACTOR

Cervix normally acts as a sperm reservoir. When cervical mucus is hostile, sperm storage and travel to the tube through the uterus becomes difficult. Cervical factor is mostly affected due to multiple D and C (dilatation and curettage). Previous surgery on cervix, such as cauterization, conization, or Fothergill's surgery, also disturbs cervical environment. As these operations are extremely rare nowadays, cervical factor is not commonly seen as a cause of infertility. In cases with repeated negative postcoital tests, with normal semen parameters, IUI in natural cycle definitely increases the probability of conception.[11] Ovarian stimulation and IUI both independently increase pregnancy rate. So controlled ovarian stimulation, even in cervical factor should be used to improve pregnancy rate.

IMMUNOLOGICAL FACTOR

Superovulation with IUI should be offered as first line of treatment in male immunological infertililty.[12]

How does immunological infertility occur?

At birth, spermatozoa are not present and so body does not recognize sperms by immune system. Sperms appear at the time of puberty and produce lot of proteins. But, because of blood testes barrier, these do not come in contact with the immune system. So, antisperm antibodies are not normally produced. But, immunological infertility is common after vasectomy, torsion, varicocele, trauma, orchitis, testicular biopsy, and even blunt injuries that break the blood-testis barrier and expose the sperm protein to blood.

Intrauterine insemination is the first choice in these cases and four cycles of IUI should be tried before IVF.[12] Steroids are not recommended nowadays, as results of IUI are better than steroid therapy.[13] Addition of 2% albumin in buffering media is useful to prevent agglutination of sperms and pregnancy rates are higher than that with steroids. Addition of chymotrypsin also helps.[14]

Agglutination is the screening test for diagnosis of immunological infertility and then confirmation is done with other tests. Mixed antiglobulin reaction (MAR) test and immunobead test are useful. Sperm immobilization test only detects IgG antibodies. IgA antibodies are more harmful. The mechanism of ASAs (antisperm antibodies) interfering with conception is disturbance of sperm transport, gamete interaction, acrosome reaction, zona binding, and pronuclear formation. If >50% of sperms are bound to antibodies, cervical penetration is markedly decreased and so is motility. If >80% sperms are bound to antibodies, then intracytoplasmic sperm injection (ICSI) is recommended.

Tung et al. postulated that small amount of spermatozoal antigen constantly leaks from epididymis and VAS activating suppressor T-lymphocytes that inhibit immune response. So under normal circumstances, ASAs are not generated.[15]

Antisperm antibodies can be suspected in cases of:

- Aggregation of sperms
- Asthenospermia
- Clinical risk of immunological infertility
- Unexplained infertility

SINGLE TUBE

In patients with one fallopian tube blocked, it is a common scenario that the follicle develops on the side on which the tube to ovary is not open.

Should we do IUI or not?

At the time of ovulation, ovarian fimbria contracts. As it is attached to ovary, the fimbrial end comes closer to the ovary and completely covers the ovarian surface at the site of the follicle. The ciliary movement of the columnar epithelium of the fallopian tube creates negative pressure of 1 mm of mercury. This negative pressure sucks the ova inside the tube. So, it is the tube that takes an ova rather than ova going inside the tube. So for successful IUI, tubo-ovarian relations should be normal and the ova enters the tube of the same side. Therefore, IUI should be done, if the tube is open on the side on which follicle develops. Sometimes, ova may be released in peritoneal cavity, if the tube is not nearby. The fimbrial end of opposite tube may capture the ova, but it is a rare incidence and here incidence of ectopic pregnancy is high.

FROZEN SAMPLE INTRAUTERINE INSEMINATION

Many a time, husband is not available at the time of IUI. So, we freeze the semen sample on the day convenient to the husband, to be utilized on the day of IUI. This is quite commonly done in today's era when the business travels or long hours working has markedly increased. If the husband is suffering from malignancy or a disease that may require chemotherapy or radiotherapy, then also semen may be cryopreserved and used on the day of IUI or ART.

HIV-DISCORDANT MALE

Intrauterine insemination is safe, effective, and less expensive option for avoiding transmission in HIV-discordant couples, where male partner is HIV positive.[16] However, some clinics recommend polymerase chain reaction (PCR) testing of the wash sample.

DONOR SPERMS

This is the option required in cases of:

- Azoospermia
- Severe oligozoospermia
- Males with genetic disorders
- Lesbian couples
- Single mother
- Failed IVF in socioeconomically weak and poor patients

Artificial insemination of donor sperms (AID) with IUI should always be given the option before taking the patient for ART. Many patients cannot afford ART, but they can still earn the joy of parenthood with AID and may also positively opt for it.

SEXUAL DISORDERS

- Hypospadias
- Retrograde ejaculation
- Impotence

- Premature ejaculation
- Vaginismus
- Neurological problems

CARRY HOME MESSAGE

- Intrauterine insemination is the first line of treatment for unexplained infertility.
- Ovulation dysfunction patients are treated by IUI.
- Improve sperm count and convert IVF cycle into IUI cycle.
- IUI is a treatment of choice in first- and second-degree endometriosis.
- In immunological infertility, IUI is useful.
- In couples with HIV-positive male partner, IUI is safe.

REFERENCES

1. Verhulst SM, Cohlen BJ, Hughes E, te Velde E, Heineman MJ. Intrauterine insemination for unexplained subfertility. Cochrane Database Syst Rev. 2006;(4):CD005356.
2. Wessel JA, Mochtar MH, Besselink DE, Betjes H, deBruin JP, Cantineau AEP, et al. Expectant management versus IUI in unexplained subfertility and a poor pregnancy prognosis (EXIUI study): a randomized controlled trial. Hum Reprod. 2022;37(12):2808-16.
3. Chiu YH, Yland JJ, Rinaudo P, Hsu J, McGrath S, Hernandez-Diaz S, et al. Effectiveness and safety of intrauterine insemination vs. assisted reproductive technology: emulating a target trial using and observational database of administrative claims. Fertil Steril. 2022; 117(5):981-91.
4. Guzick DS, Carson SA, Coutifaris C, Overstreet JW, Factor-Litvak P, Steinkampf MP, et al. Efficacy of superovulation and intra-uterine insemination in treatment of infertility. National co-operative reproductive medicine network. N Engl J Med. 1999;340(3):177-83.
5. Veltman-Verhulst SM, Hughes E, Ayeleke R, Cohlen BJ. Intrauterine insemination for unexplained infertility. Cochrane Database Syst Rev. 2016;(2):CD001838.
6. Van Ruste MM, Custers IM, Van der Veen F, van Wely M, Evers JLH, Mol BWJ. The influence of number of follicles on pregnancy rates in intrauterine insemination with ovarian stimulation: a meta-analysis. Hum Reprod Update. 2008;14(6):563-70.
7. World Health organization. Laboratory annual for the examination of Human Semen and Semen-cervical mucus interaction, 5th edition. New York: Cambridge University Press; 2010. p. 287.
8. Van Weert JM, Repping S, Van Voorhis BJ, Van der Veen F, Bossyut P, Mol BW. Performance of post-wash total motile sperm count as a predictor of pregnancy at the time of intrauterine insemination: a meta-analysis. Fertil Steril. 2004;82(3):612-20.
9. Ghanem ME, Bakre NI, Enam MA, Al Boghdady LA, Helal AS, Elmetwally AG, et al. The effect of timing of IUI in relation to ovulation and number of inseminations on cycle pregnancy rate in common infertility etiology. Hum Reprod. 2011;26(3):576-83.
10. Royal College of Obstetricians and Gynecologists (RCOG). The investigation and management of endometriosis. London (UK): Royal College of Obstetricians and Gynecologists (RCOG); 2006. p. 14. (Green-top guideline no. 24).
11. Steures P, Van der Steeg JW, Hompes PG, Bossuyt PM, Habbema JD, Eijkemans MJ, et al. Effectiveness of intrauterine insemination in subfertile couples with an isolated cervical factor: a randomized clinical trial. Fertil Steril. 2007;88(6):1692-96.
12. Ombelet W, Vandeput H, Jansen M, Cox A, Vossen C, Pollet H, et al. Treatment of male infertility due to sperm surface antibodies: IUI or IVF? Hum Reprod. 1997;12(6):1165-70.
13. Lähteenmäki Am Veilahti J, Hovatta O. Intrauterine insemination versus cyclic, low dose prednisolone in couples with male antisperm antibodies. Hum Reprod. 1995;10(1): 142-7.
14. Check JH, Hourani W, Check ML, Graziano V, Levin E. Effect of treating antibody-coated sperm with chymotrypsin on pregnancy rates following IUI as compared outcome to IVF/ICSI. Arch Androl. 2004;50(2):93-5.
15. Tung KSK. Autoimmunity of testis. In: Dhinsa DS, Schumacher GFB (Eds). Immunological aspects of infertility and fertility regulation. New York: Elsevier North Holland. 1980.
16. Vitorino R, Grinsztejn B, Ferreira de Andrade C, Hökerberg Y. Systematic review of effectiveness and safety of assisted reproduction techniques in couples serodiscordant for human immuno-deficiency virus where the man is positive. Fertil Steril. 2004;95(5):1684-90.

CHAPTER 4

Ultrasound Monitoring of IUI Cycle

INTRODUCTION

Ultrasound is the modality of choice for monitoring of the patients on ovulation induction for intrauterine insemination (IUI) cycles. When used with Doppler, it gives precise idea not only about the morphological changes but also about the hormonal changes occurring during the entire cycle, because the hormonal changes first reflect as vascular changes and then as morphological changes. Therefore, if vascular changes are observed with Doppler, the need of hormonal assessments for cycle monitoring can be omitted.

The discussion about of the role of ultrasound during the entire treatment cycle will be divided into three parts:

1. Baseline scan and deciding the stimulation protocol
2. Preovulatory scan and decision on trigger
3. Luteal phase scan

BASELINE SCAN AND DECIDING THE STIMULATION PROTOCOL

This scan is done on Day 2–3 of the menstrual cycle. The ovaries are silent and have no active follicle or corpus luteum at this stage. Route of scan has to be transvaginal always to allow better resolution and more anatomical details of ovary and endometrium. All the scans are done using B-mode ultrasound with color Doppler, pulse Doppler. 3D ultrasound and 3D power Doppler may be added in cases of doubt.

The decision on stimulation protocol or doses of gonadotropins to be used for ovulation induction are dependent on this scan reports. The scan is done to assess ovarian reserve and ovarian response. Ovarian reserve means likely number of follicles that may develop on ovulation induction, and this depends on antral follicle count (AFC) and ovarian volume. Ovarian response indicates approximate doses that would be required to produce one or more mature follicles. This depends on the ovarian stromal flow. If the blood flow to the ovary is abundant, gonadotropins will reach ovary in large amount and, therefore, total drugs required to be injected into patient's system will be less. Whereas, if blood flow to ovary is scanty, total chemical delivered to the ovary will be a smaller fragment of whatever is loaded into patient's system. Therefore, to allow sufficient amount of drugs to reach ovary, larger amounts must be put into patient's system. The total blood flow to the ovarian stroma can be judged by the resistance in the blood vessels and the peak systolic velocity (PSV) of the blood flow in these vessels. Blood flow resistance is assessed by an index called resistance index (RI). The antral follicle count and ovarian stromal flow parameters on the baseline scan are shown to be most predictive of the ovarian response after pituitary downregulation in a study, followed by total ovarian volume, ovarian stromal area, and age.[1]

According to another study[2] also, total number of antral follicles and ovarian stromal blood flow were the two most significant predictors of ovarian response and ovarian volume was highly significant predictor of number of follicles and oocytes retrieved. The results of this study were in absolute favor of individualizing dose according to the dosage nomogram proving the reliability of ultrasound parameters and age and BMI for decision on stimulation doses. An ultrasound-based study on prediction of ovarian response in 2007 by Merce et al.[3] evaluated ovarian volume, AFC, and 3D power Doppler indices VI (vascularization index), FI (flow index), and VFI (vascularity flow index) for their reliability to calculate the number of follicles grown, oocyte retrieved, and embryos transferred. This study clearly showed the relevance of ovarian volume and AFC to the number of follicles matured and oocytes retrieved. It also mentioned that 3D power Doppler indices made the assessment of ovarian response to stimulation protocols easier.

The parameters that we have used to calculate the dose for gonadotropins stimulation protocol for IUI cycles in our study are—age, BMI, AFC, ovarian volume, stromal RI, and PSV.

Antral follicle count showed the best correlation with women's age and declined linearly at a rate of 3.8% per year.[4]

Is AFC sufficient as a measure of ovarian reserve or AMH (anti-Müllerian hormone) required?

Linear correlation is seen between AFC and AMH and both help to predict the extremes of response. AMH and AFC both have reflections of primordial follicles, and both are stable between cycles.[5] Antral follicle count and ovarian volume showed significant correlation with AMH.[6] Serum AMH levels have been shown to strongly correlate with the number of antral follicles.[7] For prediction of poor ovarian response, a model including AFC + AMH was found to be almost similar to that of (*p value*: 0.001) using AFC alone.[8] In a meta-analysis by Broer et al., it has been shown that AMH has at least the same level of accuracy and clinical value for the prediction of poor response and nonpregnancy as AFC.[9] AFC and AMH have been shown to be equally accurate for predicting ovarian reserve in normal reserve ovaries and polycystic ovaries.[10] Doing AFC assessment alone would be more cost-effective for predicting the ovarian response in patients undergoing controlled ovarian stimulation.

Moreover, for IUI cycles, maximum 2–3 follicles need to grow to maturity and a low ovarian reserve does not matter much. AFC can be used to predict multifollicular growth and gonadotropin doses can be controlled accordingly.

Precise calculation of AFC, therefore, can help in predicting the ovarian response. This can be done on 2D ultrasound or by 3D with sono-AVC (automated volume calculation), a specialized 3D ultrasound software for calculation of antral follicle number and volumes. This method is more precise, as there is least chance of follicles being missed or being counted twice because of color coding. But, postprocessing is required for accurate calculations. It takes longer to perform, because of the need for postprocessing, and obtains values that are lower than those obtained by the 2D and 3D-MPV techniques[11,12] **(Fig. 1)**. But, as long as the number of follicles is 12–15 per ovary, both 2D and 3D ultrasound can be equally reliable.[13] On 2D ultrasound, the AFC can be calculated by scrolling through both the ovaries one by one and eyeball and count the number of antral follicles.

Antral follicle count and ovarian volume provide direct measurements of ovarian reserve.[14]

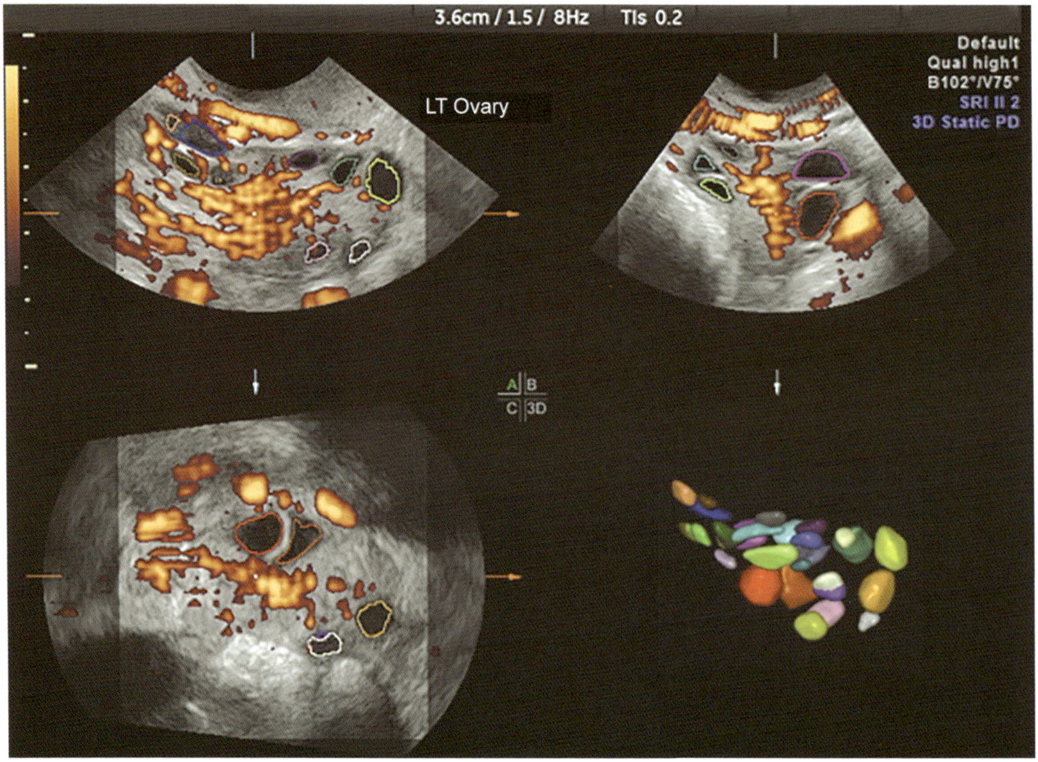

Fig. 1: 3D ultrasound of the ovary with sono-automated volume calculation (AVC) for calculating antral follicle counts.

Ovarian volume <3 cc was significantly predictive of higher IVF cancellation rates (>50%)[15] **(Fig. 2)**. Though is included in our scoring system for deciding stimulation doses, it is not of much importance as far as IUI cycles are concerned because multifollicular development is not required here. On the contrary, ovarian volume assessment in IUI cycles on baseline is required to be careful not to increase the gonadotropin doses to too high. It can be measured by 2D ultrasound by measuring three orthogonal diameters or by 3D by using a software called virtual organ computer-aided analysis (VOCAL). Once ovary is located, the probe is rotated to find out the longest diameter of ovary and is stored as one frame on a dual screen. Then the probe is rotated 90° to get a true transverse axis of ovary. Measure the largest longitudinal, transverse, and anteroposterior (AP) diameter of the ovary in centimeters (cm), and ovarian volume can be calculated by the formula ($x \times y \times z \times 0.523$).

Age is known to be one of the most important factors that reduce not only the ovarian reserve but also the oocyte quality. The ovarian stromal blood flow was found to be negatively correlated with age. It has been shown in several studies above-mentioned that BMI may be an important determinant of the ovarian response. This is because flow in the ovarian stroma is less in obese patients as compared to controls.[5]

Stromal blood flow is one of the decision-making parameters. It has been shown that measurement of ovarian stromal flow in early follicular phase is related to subsequent ovarian response.[16]

Ovarian stromal PSV after pituitary suppression is predictive of ovarian responsiveness.[17] Ovarian blood flow predicts ovarian responsiveness and hence provides a non-

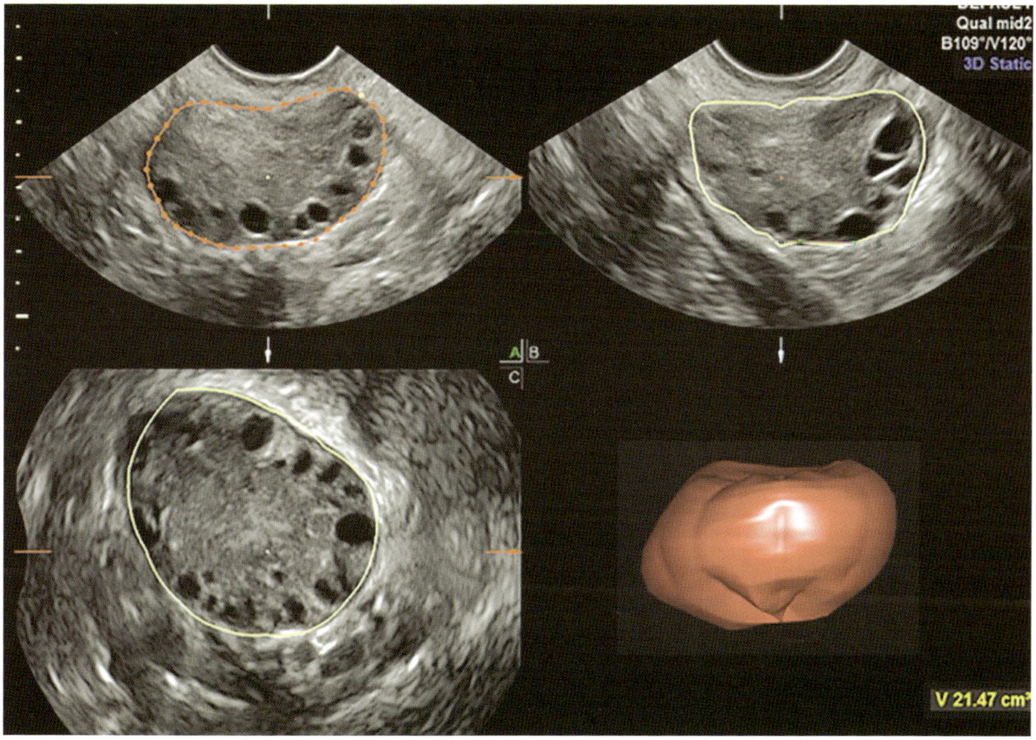

Fig. 2: 3D ultrasound calculated ovarian volume by a software called virtual organ computer-aided analysis (VOCAL).

invasive and cost-effective prognostic factor of response to ovarian stimulation.[18]

Based on all these facts and findings, it is understood that for ovaries that have high resistance, low-velocity flow **(Fig. 3)** requires higher doses of gonadotropins for stimulation; whereas, those with low resistance, high-velocity flow **(Fig. 4)** requires lower doses of gonadotropins for stimulation.

The final dose calculation can be based on the above-discussed factors, and a scoring system was developed based on clinical and ultrasound findings as given in **Table 1**.[19]

Based on the scores of individual patient, calculated as in **Table 1**, the gonadotropin (rFSH) doses were individualized as mentioned in **Table 2** for IUI cycles.[19]

As per the results of our study, it is indicated that stimulation doses that calculated from the baseline score, are highly reliable for safe planning of stimulation protocols in IUI cycles, as the OHSS rates and cycle cancellation rates due to poor response are negligible. Multiple pregnancy rates are also acceptable. This study we believe may prove to be an important guide for safe use of gonadotropins for ovulation induction in ART cycles.[19]

The same scoring system and the dose calculation can be used for only gonadotropin (rFSH) or letrozole + rFSH protocols. Though the doses for urinary products and human menopausal gonadotropins need to be modified. As mentioned in the chapter on stimulation protocols for IUI in this book, we prefer to use either rFSH or highly purified FSH only for IUI cycles.

As mentioned in the same chapter, in letrozole + gonadotropin protocol, gonadotropin is started on Day 7/8 of cycle after letrozole and for gonadotropin alone cycle, gonadotropin is started on Day 5. Scan is always done on the Day, gonadotropin is started. If there is a follicle of larger than 10 mm, patient is called back when the

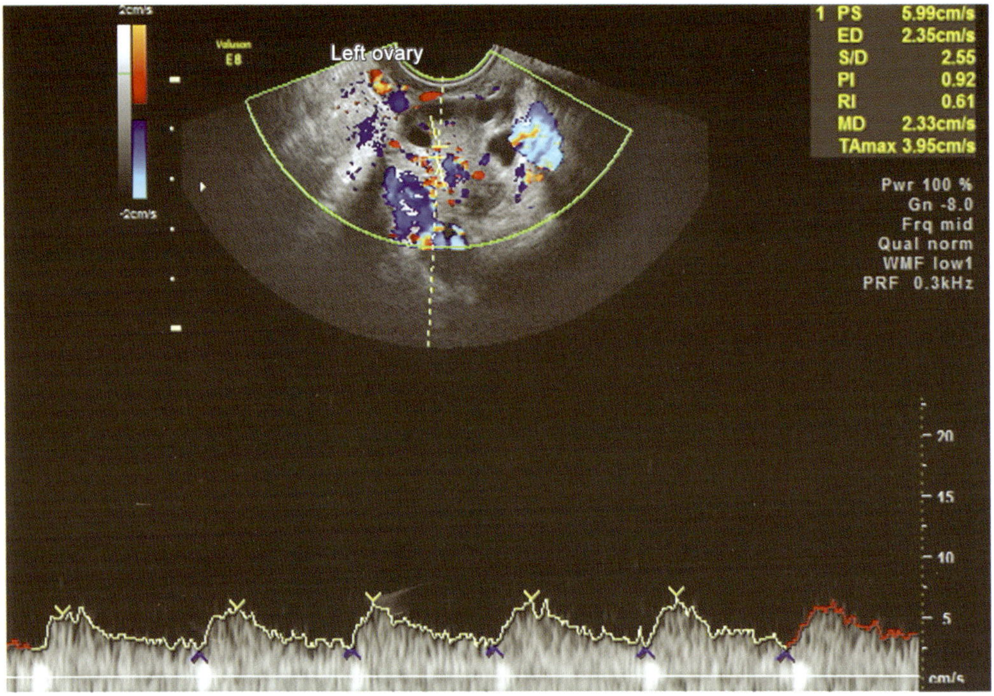

Fig. 3: Ovarian stromal flow as seen on color Doppler and pulse Doppler.

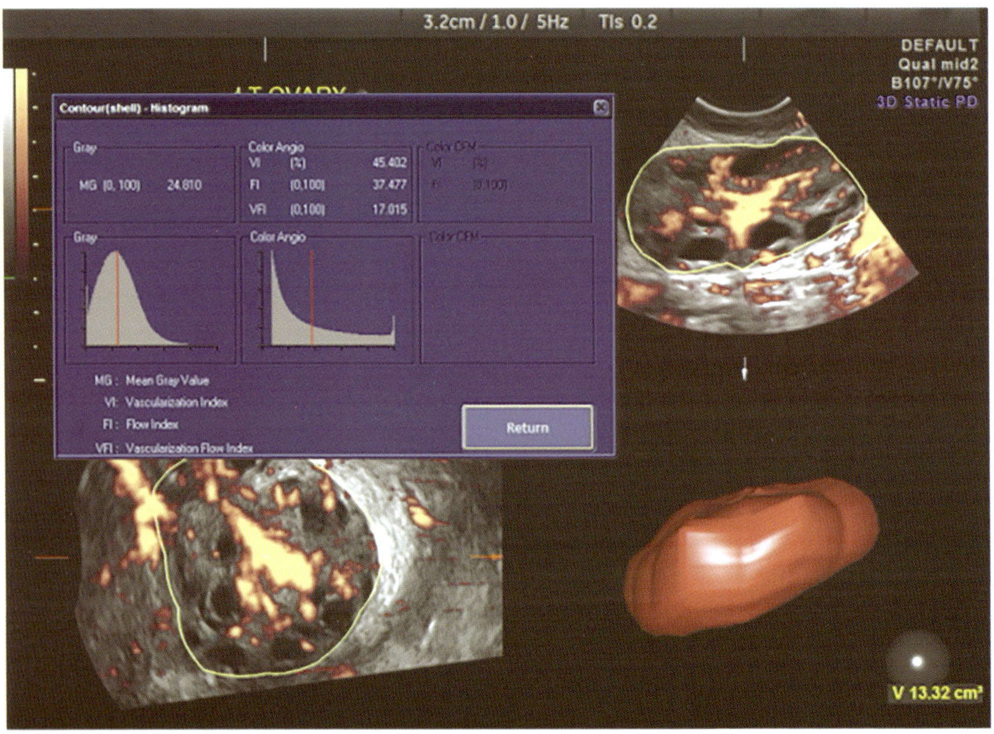

Fig. 4: 3D power Doppler ultrasound with virtual organ computer-aided analysis (VOCAL) calculated volume with volume histogram (blue box) showing vascularity index (VI), flow index (FI), and vascularity flow index (VFI) parameters.

TABLE 1: Baseline scoring system.[19]

Score	***1***	***2***	***3***	***4***	***5***
Age	>40	35.1–40	30.1–35	25.1–30	<25
BMI	>30	30–28.1	28–25.1	25–22.1	<22
AFC	<5	5–10	10–15	15–20	>20
Ovary volume	<3	3.1–5	5.1–7	7.1–10	>10
Stromal RI	>0.75	0.75–0.66	0.65–0.56	0.55–0.45	<0.45
Stromal PSV	<3	3.1–5	5.1–7	7.1–10	>10

(AFC: antral follicle count; BMI: body mass index; RI: resistance index; PSV: peak systolic velocity)

TABLE 2: Dose of recombinant follicle-stimulating hormone (rFSH) according to baseline score.[19]

Score	***Dose***
>25	25 IU
20–24	37.5
15–20	75 IU
10–15	112.5 IU
6–10	150 IU

follicle is likely to reach 18 mm. This can be estimated because a follicle that is of >10 mm in diameter is a dominant follicle and it grows at a rate of 2–3 mm per day. It has no internal echogenicity and has thin (pencil line like) walls, is not only more likely to become the leading follicle but will also give mature healthy ovum. If all the follicles are smaller than 10 mm on the Day gonadotropin is started, the patient is called after 5 days. As the dominant follicle grows, it starts pulling vascularity toward itself.[16,17]

B-mode Features of a Mature Follicle

The follicular diameter is measured when the follicle is seen as a rounded structure, or three orthogonal diameters must be measured and the mean is used as follicular diameter. A mature follicle is 16–18 mm **(Fig. 5)**, has thin walls, regular round shape, and no echogenicity in the lumen, and shows a thin hypoechoic rim surrounding the follicle and sometimes (about 35–40%) cumulus-like shadow may be seen. This thin hypoechoic rim and cumulus-like shadow develops approximately 36 hours before rupture. A flimsy irregular line is seen inside the follicle parallel to the wall about 6–10 hours before rupture **(Fig. 6)**.

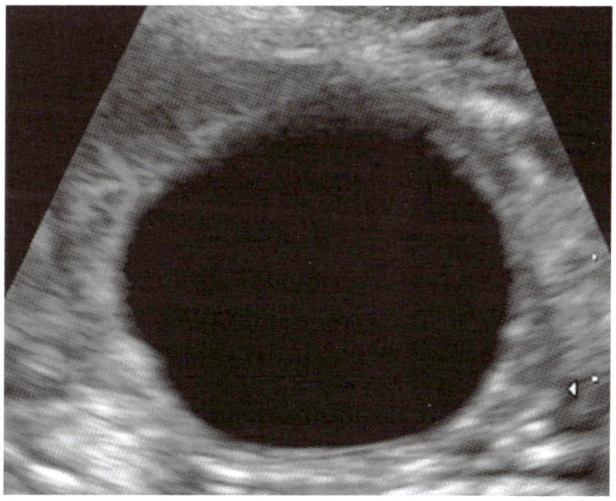

Fig. 5: B-mode ultrasound image of a mature follicle.

Doppler Features of a Good Preovulatory Follicle

Increase in perifollicular vascularity of dominant follicle in theca layer starts developing as early as 8th day of the cycle. Fall in perifollicular RI starts 2 days before ovulation, reaches nadir at ovulation, remains low for 4 days and then with gradual rise reaches 0.5 in mid luteal phase.[20]

When functionally mature, on color Doppler, the follicle shows blood vessels covering at least 3/4th of the follicular

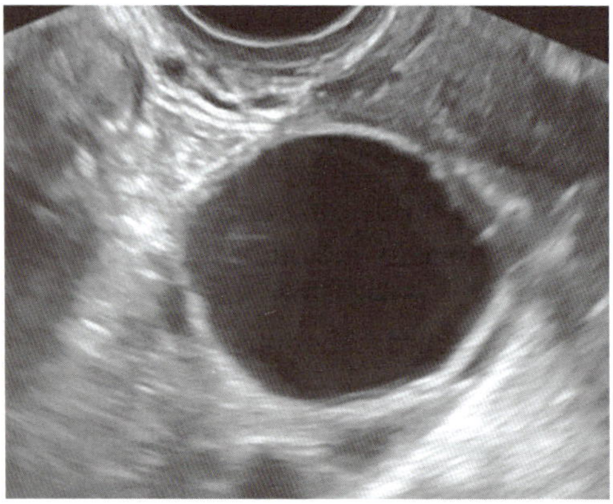

Fig. 6: B-mode ultrasound image of a follicle of which rupture is impending showing mild separation of inner wall at 2 o' clock and 6 o' clock positions.

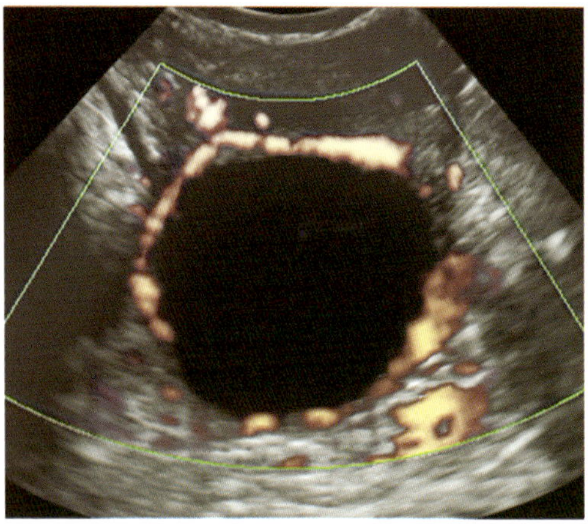

Fig. 7: Perifollicular vascularity seen on color Doppler.

circumference **(Fig. 7)**. Chui et al. graded the follicular flow on the day of oocyte collection as grade 1–4 when in a single cross area slice the flow covered <25%, 25–50%, 50–75%, >75% of follicular circumference. The conception was related to grade 3–4 vascularity.[21]

On pulse Doppler, these blood vessels show RI of 0.4–0.48[21] and PSV of >10 cm/s **(Fig. 8)**.

The pulse repetition frequency (PRF) settings for color Doppler are set at 0.3 and wall filter at the lowest. The perifollicular vessels are only those that obliterate the follicular wall with color. If the follicular wall is seen and the vessel is seen just besides it, it is not a perifollicular vessel. Ovarian flow correlates well with oocyte recovery rates and, hence, may be useful in determining the most appropriate time to administer ovulation trigger to optimize recovery rate. It has been quoted in a study by Nargund et al.[21,22] that embryos produced by fertilization of the ova obtained from the follicles, that had a perifollicular PSV of <10 cm/s, are less likely to be grade 1 embryos and also have higher chance of chromosomal malformations. In the same study, it has been shown that the probability of developing a grade 1 or 2 embryo is 75%, if PSV was >10 cm/s, 40%, if PSV was <10 cm/s, 24%, if there was no perifollicular flow. There is yet another study that supports this finding. Oocytes from severely hypoxic follicles are associated with high frequency of abnormalities of organization of chromosomes on metaphase spindle and may lead to segregation disorders and catastrophic mosaics in embryo.[23]

On 3D ultrasound, the follicular volume of 3–7.5 cc has been found to be optimum in our study.[24] This agrees with the study by Wittmack et al.,[25] which says that—in IVF-ET cycles, follicles with mean follicular diameter of 12–24 mm are associated with optimal rates of oocyte recovery, fertilization, and cleavage.[25] This corresponds to the follicular volumes of between 3 and 7 mL. The accuracy of 3D US measurement of follicular volume compared to the standard 2D techniques by comparing the volume of individual follicles estimated by both methods, 3D ultrasound with VOCAL gave much more accurate measurements[26] **(Fig. 9)**.

It has been shown that follicular fluid concentrations of leptin, a follicular angiogenesis-related factor, are inversely related to the stromal blood flow index.[27]

It has also been suggested that the follicles containing oocytes capable to produce a pregnancy have a perifollicular vascular network more uniform and distinctive.[28]

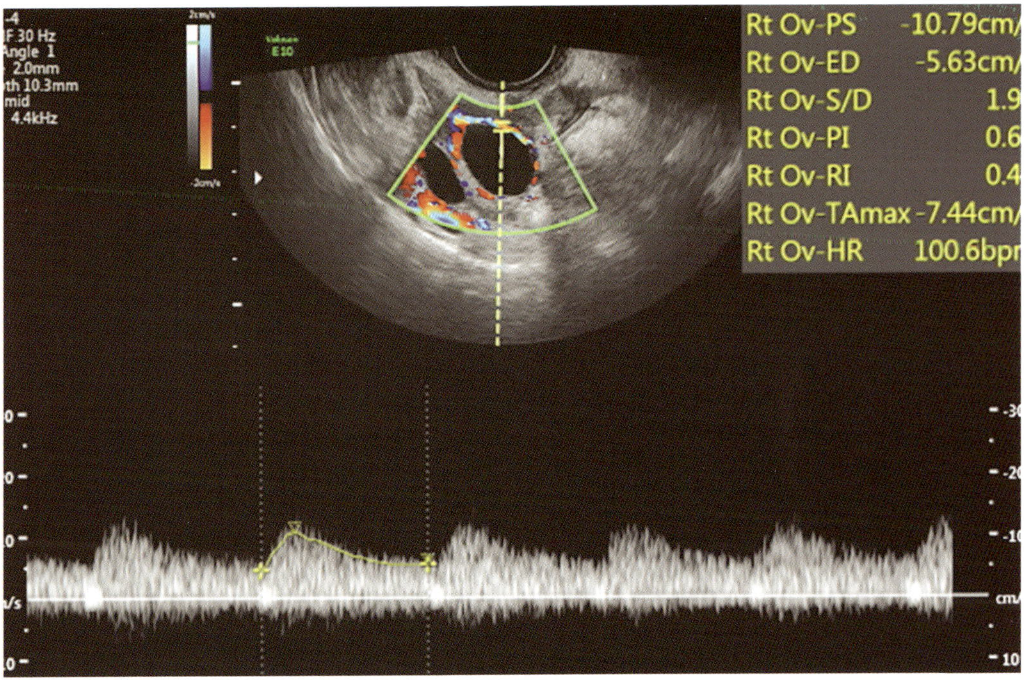

Fig. 8: Pulse Doppler of the low-resistance perifollicular flow.

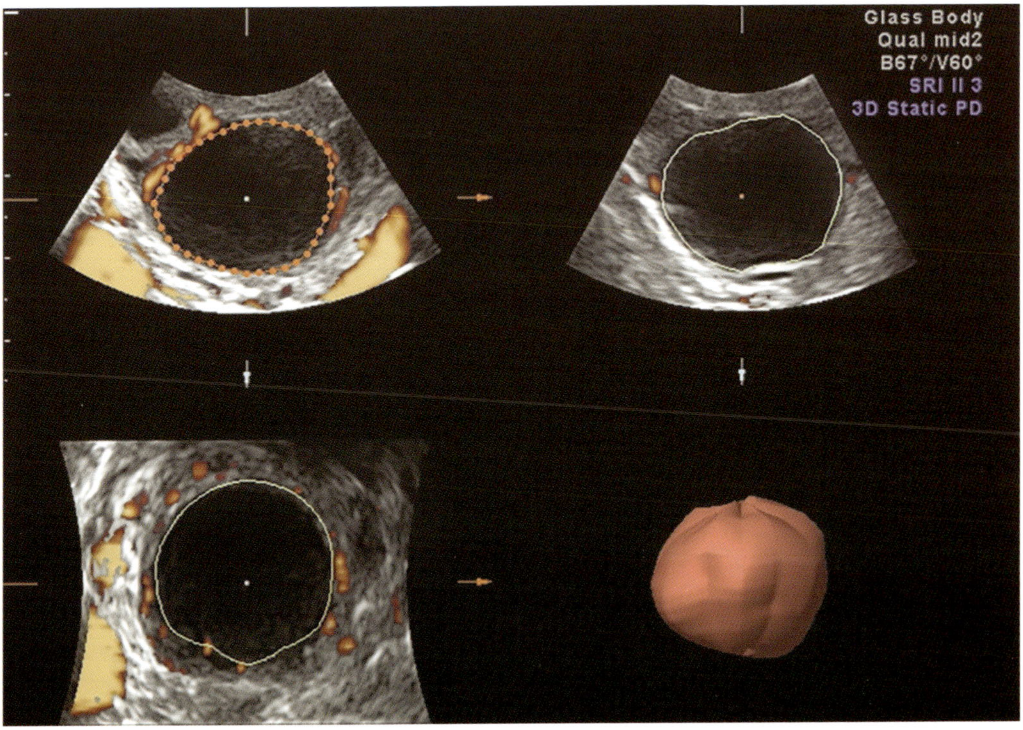

Fig. 9: 3D ultrasound acquired virtual organ computer-aided analysis (VOCAL) calculated volume of follicle.

In our study,[24] we have found perifollicular VI of between 6 and 20 and perifollicular FI >35 as most optimum. 68.4% of patients conceived when the VI was between 6 and 18 and 50% when it was between 18 and 20. However, the pregnancy rates were <25%, when VI was <6 and only 7.4%, when VI was >20. It was only 7.4% of patients with FI <27 who conceived, whereas beyond 27, the conception rates rose consistently. It was 50% with FI between 27 and 35, 70% when FI was between 35 and 43 and almost all patients had conceived when FI was >43. Although it is possible to assess the follicular flow as expressed by the peak systolic velocity and perifollicular color map,[29] it is the 3D power Doppler that gives the most precise information about the vascularization and follicular blood flow.[30] Trigger plays a major role in inducing influx of blood within follicles. At the LH surge, the perifollicular PSV is 10 cm/s.

This means that if the follicle is said to be functionally mature when PSV is 10 cm/s, that is the time when the LH surge starts and under the effect of that LH, the perifollicular PSV keeps on rising constantly.[31] This derives that a rising PSV with steady low RI suggests that the follicle is close to rupture. Vascular changes at the time of impending ovulation include increased vascularity of the inner wall of the follicle and a coincident surge in blood velocity just prior to eruption.[31] Our unpublished study of 350 IUI cycles has shown that when the perifollicular PSV was >20 cm/s, double IUI at 12–14 hours after trigger and 36–38 hours after trigger has given much higher pregnancy rates as compared to single IUI at 36–38 hours after trigger (presented at ISUOG, 2006). The study has also been mentioned in the chapter on timing of IUI in this book.

There are many centers where Doppler is not used or is not available. It has been documented in studies from these centers that ovulation trigger when the lead follicle is 21–22 mm is associated with higher odds of clinical pregnancy in patients undergoing first CC-IUI for the ovulatory dysfunction of unexplained infertility.[32]

This higher clinical pregnancy rate is due to higher E2. This higher E2 will counteract anti-estrogen action of CC on endometrium.

Implantation has been the weakest link in the success of infertility treatment. Endometrium is a receptor organ for majority of the hormones involved in fertility and, therefore, study of its morphology and vascularity is thought to explain the mysteries of implantation failure. Therefore, like follicle, endometrium is also assessed by transvaginal 2D US and color Doppler before planning for trigger during any assisted reproductive technologies.

B-mode Features of Endometrium with Good Receptivity

On transvaginal sonography (TVS), an endometrial thickness of minimum 6 mm is required on the day of trigger, but 8–10 mm is optimum. Endometrial thickness has more negative predictive value for implantation. Morphology of the endometrium is as important as thickness of the endometrium. In all the healthy endometria, the endometrial-myometrial interface is always seen as a clear hypoechoic halo surrounding the whole endometrium **(Fig. 10)**. Breach or irregularity

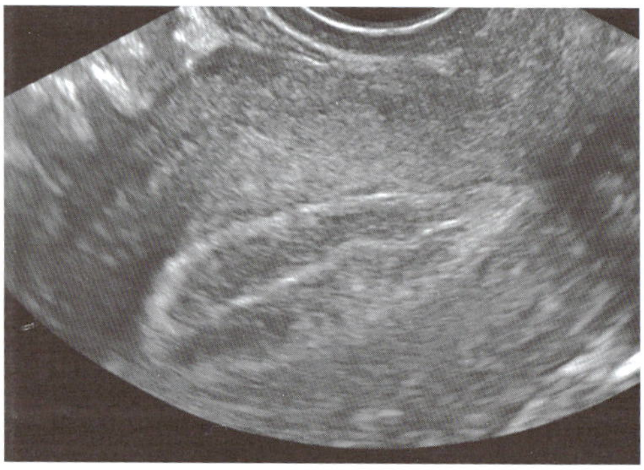

Fig. 10: B-mode ultrasound of grade A endometrium with intact endometriomyometrial junction.

of endometrial-myometrial junction is an indication of unhealthy endometrium and therefore poor receptivity.

Popularly multilayered endometrium is considered as a desired endometrial pattern. Morphologically, the endometrium is graded as the best grade A, when it is a triple line endometrium with the intervening area is as hypoechoic as the anterior myometrium. The echogenicity is attributed to the development of multiple vessels penetrating in the endometrium producing multiple tissue interfaces and therefore causing the echogenicity and due to glycogen storage in the endometrial columnar epithelium **(Fig. 11)**. The endometrium is graded as intermediate or grade B **(Fig. 12)**, when it is multilayered or triple line with hypoechoic intervening area. In grade C, the endometrium is homogeneous isoechoic endometrium.[33] Though some studies have shown no significant difference in pregnancy rates among different morphological patterns. According to literature evidence and our experience, different morphological patterns of the endometrium can be related to the estradiol levels. As estradiol level increases, the endometrium becomes triple line, increases in thickness, and progresses from grade B to grade A, and then to grade C with supraphysiological levels of estradiol as occurs in multifollicular development.

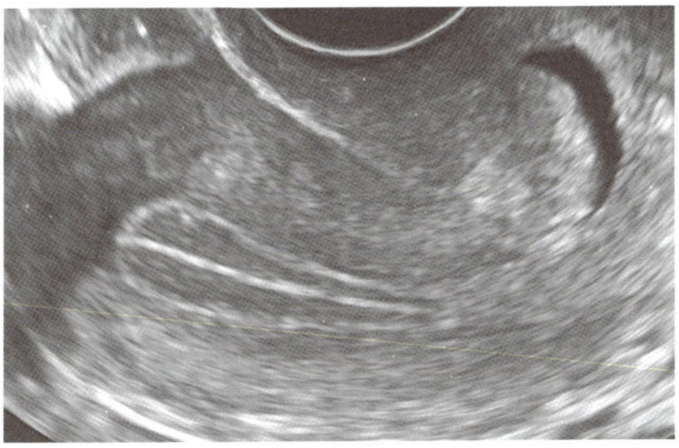

Fig. 11: B-mode ultrasound of grade B endometrium.

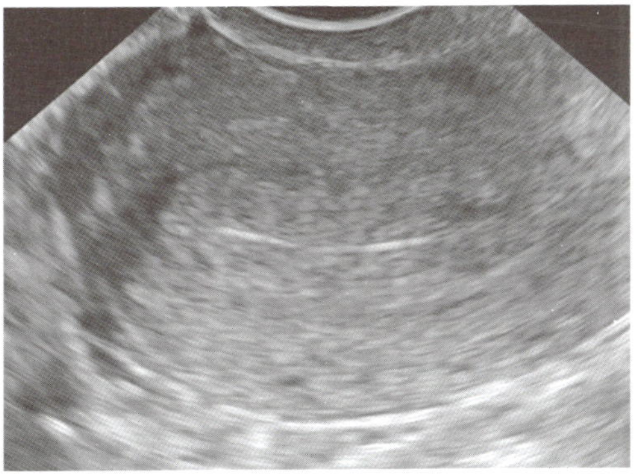

Fig. 12: B-mode ultrasound of grade C endometrium.

Doppler Features of Endometrium with Good Receptivity

There are several reports by different groups[34] that agree on the fact that implantation rates can be more correlated to the vascularity of the endometrium rather than the thickness and morphology of the endometrium.

Segmental uterine artery perfusion demonstrates significant correlation with hormonal and histological markers of uterine receptivity, reaching the highest sensitivity for subendometrial blood flow. On color Doppler, the endometrium, which is mature, shows vascularity in zone 3 and 4 or may be called subendometrial and endometrial layers **(Fig. 13)**.

The zones of vascularity are defined according to Applebaum[34] as—zone 1 when the vascularity on power Doppler is seen only at endometrial-myometrial junction, Zone 2 when vessels penetrate through the hyperechogenic endometrial edge, Zone 3 when it reaches intervening hypoechogenic zone and zone 4 when these reach the endometrial cavity. But, a particular zone can be called vascularized only, when at least 5 mm^2 area of that zone is vascularized. Below this cut-off for zone 3–4, the pregnancy rates are extremely low.[35]

One more comparison of two studies has also shown similar results:[36]

- *Zone 1:* 3.5–7.5%; 5.2%
- *Zone 2:* 15.8–29.7%; 28.7%

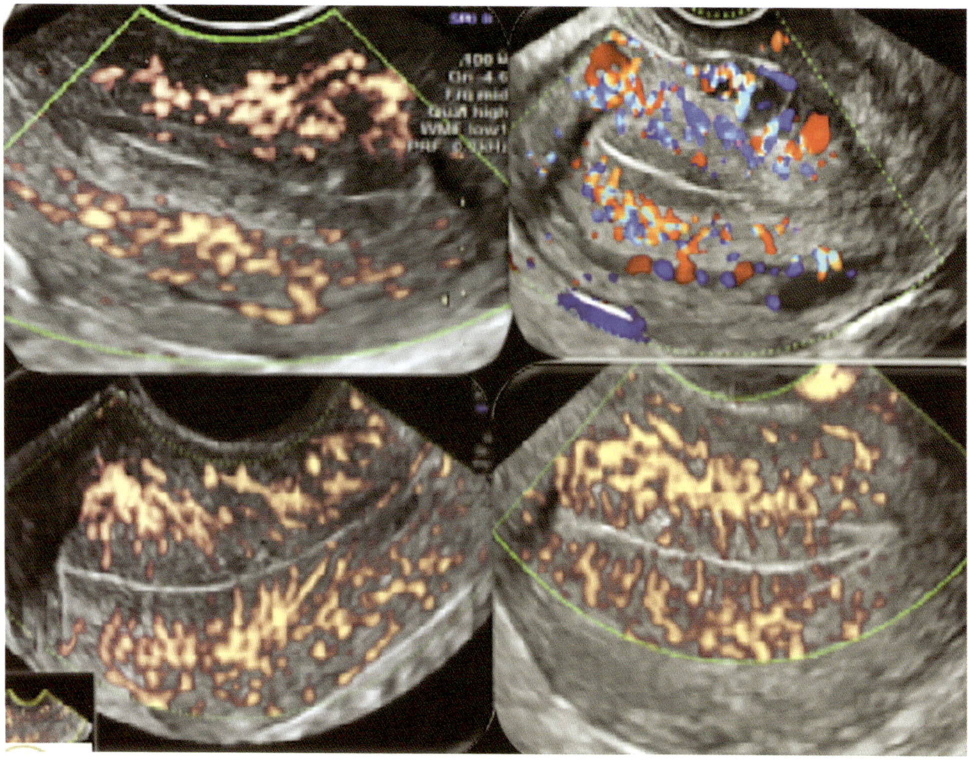

Fig. 13: Power Doppler images of the zone 1–4 endometrial vascularity.

- *Zone 3:* 24.2–47.8%; 52%
- *Zone 4:* 67.3%; 74%

Endometrial vascularity: Its relation to implantation rates (Nagori and Panchal)[37]

Vascularity in	*Zone 1*	*Zone 2*	*Zone 3*	*Zone 4*
% of patients	6.69%	20.73%	58%	14.47%
+ β-hCG	19%	21.87%	39.77%	70.14
Gestational sac	9.6%	14.58%	36.8%	68.65%
Abortions	50%	23.8%	5.6%	1.5%

Zaidi et al. found that absence of flow in the endometrial and subendometrial zones on day of trigger indicates total failure of implantation.[38]

The vessels that reach the endometrium are the spiral arteries. The pulse Doppler of these arteries should have an RI <0.6 for the endometrium to be called mature for implantation.

Moreover, the pulse Doppler analysis of the uterine artery waveform is done, and its PI should be <3.2 **(Fig. 14)**.

Several authors have shown that the optimum uterine receptivity was obtained when average pulsatility index of the uterine artery was between 2 and 3 on the day of transfer or on the day of trigger.[39,40]

Coulam et al. have also shown that no pregnancy was achieved after embryo transfer when uterine artery PI was above 3.3 in an IVF program also.[41]

Cacciatore et al. suggest that implantation is unlikely when PI is >3.3 and RI >0.95 or when no velocities are seen at the end of the diastole.[42]

In such cases, therefore in IUI cycles, hCG is withheld or postponed.

Endometrial volume by 3D US volume calculation of the endometrium may help to correlate the cycle outcome with quantitative parameter rather than endometrial thickness.[25] This is done by the software called VOCAL.

A study by Raga et al.[43] shows pregnancy and implantation rates were significantly lower when endometrial volume <2 mL, while no pregnancy was achieved when endometrial volume was <1 mL. Study by Kupesic et al. also shows no pregnancy when endometrial volume was <2 mL, or when exceeded 8 mL.[44]

To summarize ***(Table 3)****:* If these parameters are not reached, the cycle is not cancelled,

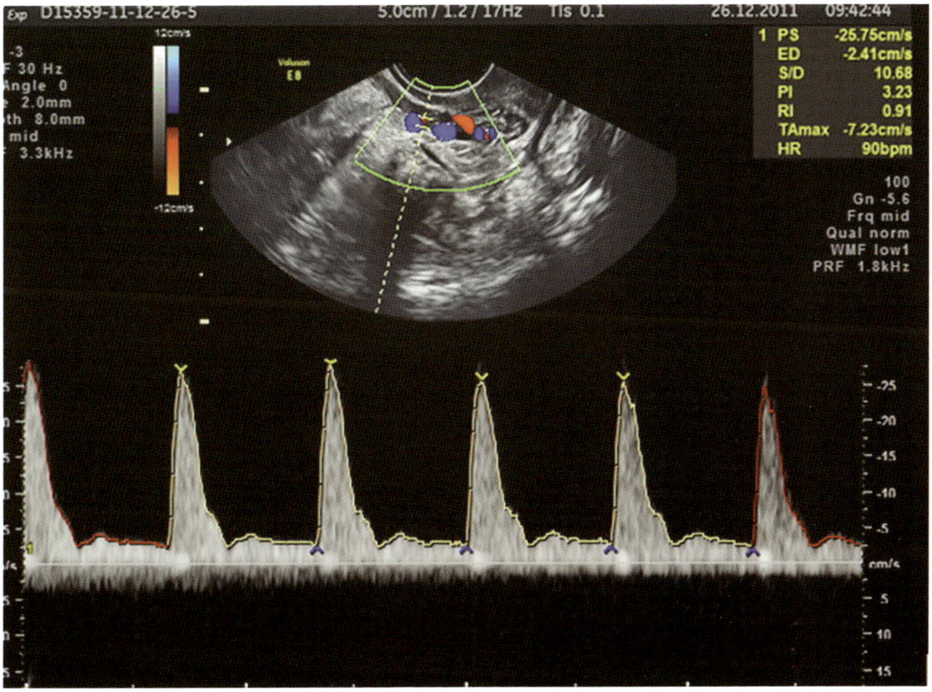

Fig. 14: Pulse Doppler showing high-resistance uterine artery flow waveform.

TABLE 3: Preovulatory follicle and endometrium.

	Follicle	***Endometrium***
Size/thickness	16–18 mm	8–10 mm
Morphology	Thin wall, no internal echoes, and halo	Grade A/B
Vascularity	3/4th circumference	Zone 3–4
RI	0.4–0.48	<0.5
PSV	>10 cm/s	—
Uterine artery PI	—	<3.2
Volume	3–7 cc	3–7 cc
3D morphology	Cumulus	Intact endometrial-myometrial junction
3D PD	More symmetrical the better	Higher the better

(PD: pulse Doppler; PI: pulsatility index; PSV: peak systolic velocity; RI: resistance index)

only delayed. Stimulation is continued till these parameters are achieved. In case, the PSV of the follicle starts rising with low RI, it means the ovulation is impending. In such a situation, in spite of inadequate endometrial parameters, trigger is given, but the patient is also explained that the results cannot be as good as it would be if every parameter was optimal. If the follicle grows beyond 23–24 mm and still perifollicular flow is not adequate, trigger is planned and patient may be given a choice of either timed intercourse or IUI, after proper explanation about the results.

Secretory Phase Assessment

Rupture of the follicle leads to formation of corpus luteum. Corpus luteum is responsible for progesterone production. The functional efficacy of the corpus luteum can be assessed by Doppler by assessing the pericorpus luteal vascularity.

Segmental uterine and ovarian artery perfusion demonstrates a significant correlation with histological and hormonal markers of uterine receptivity and may aid assessment of luteal phase defect.[45] A clear correlation between RI of corpus luteum and plasma progesterone levels has been seen in natural cycle. RI of the corpus luteum can therefore be used as an adjunct to plasma progesterone assay as an index of luteal function.[46]

A corpus luteum that is functionally normal and produces adequate amount of progesterone shows corpus luteal flow—RI 0.35–0.50 and PSV 10–15 **(Fig. 15)**.

The receptor organ for progesterone also (like estrogen) is endometrium and its vascular studies can be a reliable clue to adequate progesterone production. Though endometrial also becomes hyperechoic as a result of progesterone exposure. But soon after rupture of the follicle, the outer margin of the endometrium starts becoming fluffy and blurred. With adequate progesterone levels, that are achieved in the mid-luteal phase, the spiral arteries show RI 0.48–0.52 (low resistance flow) and uterine artery shows PI of 2.0–2.5. This PI is lower than in the preovulatory phase because of smooth muscle relaxing effect of progesterone. Inadequate progesterone production and therefore corpus luteal inadequacy is suggested by high-resistance flow in corpus luteal vessels.[46]

Whereas high-spiral artery resistance would suggest inadequate response of endometrium to progesterone. This is because of inadequate progesterone receptors in the endometrium or because of local endometrial cause, such as endometrial injury or chronic endometritis.

In luteal phase defect, because of low progesterone levels, the resistance in the

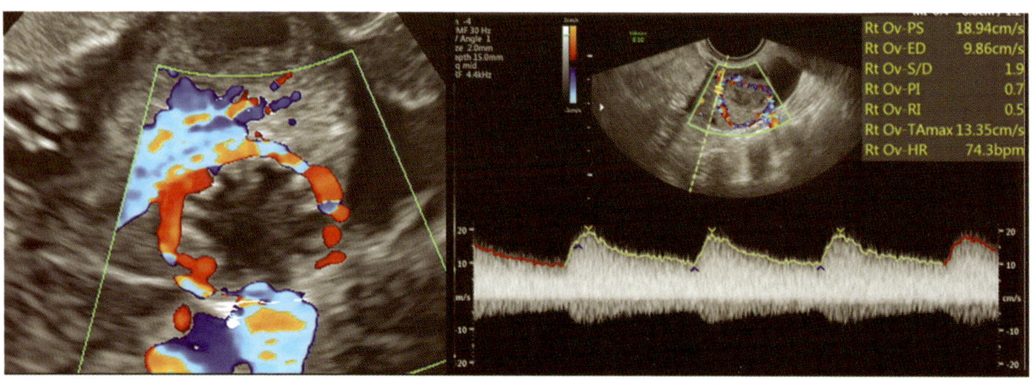

Fig. 15: Normal corpus luteal flow seen on color Doppler and pulse Doppler.

TABLE 4: Corpus luteal Doppler parameters throughout the cycle in normal cases and in luteal phase defect (LPD).

	Normal	*LPD*
Perifollicular	0.56 ± 0.06	0.58 ± 0.04
LH peak day	0.44 ± 0.04	0.58 ± 0.04
Mid-luteal phase	0.42 ± 0.06	0.58 ± 0.04
Late luteal phase	0.50 ± 0.04	0.58 ± 0.04

(LH: luteinizing hormone)

TABLE 5: Endometrial Doppler parameters throughout the cycle in normal cases and in luteal phase defect (LPD).

Phase	*Control RI*	*LPD RI*
Periovulatory	0.53 ± 0.04	0.70 ± 0.06
Mid-luteal	0.50 ± 0.02	0.72 ± 0.06
Late luteal	0.51 ± 0.04	0.72 ± 0.04

pericorpus luteal vessels is high. Because of low progesterone levels, there is inadequate relaxation of the muscularis of the uterine artery and therefore the uterine artery resistance is high along with higher resistance in its branches—the spiral vessels.

Corpus luteal flow and spiral artery flow in normal cycle and luteal phase defect[45] are mentioned in **Tables 4 and 5**.

Secretory scan is especially helpful for pinpointing the cause of failure of treatment and change the protocol, if required in the next cycle, e.g., hCG for luteal support in case of corpus luteal failure, more closer monitoring of the cycle and proper time of trigger for luteinized unruptured follicle and modification in the stimulation protocol for inadequate progesterone receptors in endometrium.

Correlation of Progesterone to Ultrasound Findings

Fluffiness of outer margin of multilayered endometrium suggests initiation of progesterone secretion **(Fig. 16)**.

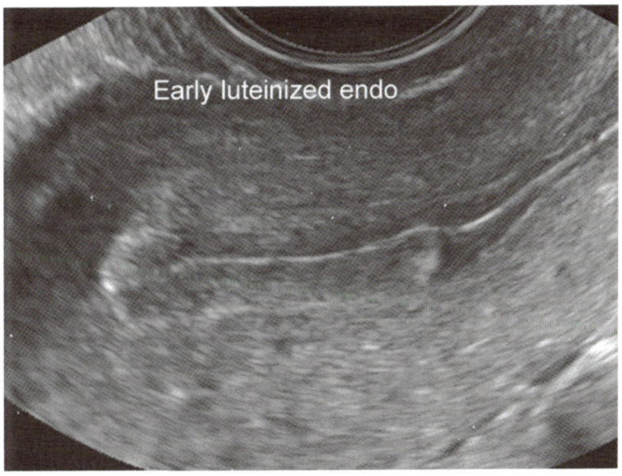

Fig. 16: Endometrium of early luteal phase seen on B-mode ultrasound. Fluffiness of outer margins of multilayered endometrium.

Low-resistance flow in corpus luteum, with echogenic endometrium **(Figs. 17A and B)** and low-resistance endometrial vascularity in mid-luteal phase, suggests normal luteal phase.

High resistance corpus luteal flow suggests corpus luteal inadequacy.

High resistance endometrial flow in mid-luteal phase suggests either inadequate progesterone levels or inadequate progesterone receptors in endometrium.

CARRY HOME MESSAGE

- Ultrasound is an excellent tool for assessment of the menstrual cycle. Hormonal changes occurring day-to-day during the menstrual cycle reflect as morphological and vascular changes in the ovary and the uterus. Assessing these changes by transvaginal ultrasound and Doppler and correctly interpreting can explain the hormonal basis of these changes. Ultrasound with Doppler can thus be used as the only modality for cycle assessment in patients undergoing assisted reproduction technology and may be of help to reduce the cost of the cycle by avoiding certain hormonal assessments and still maintaining close and accurate watch on the hormonal changes occurring during treatment cycle.

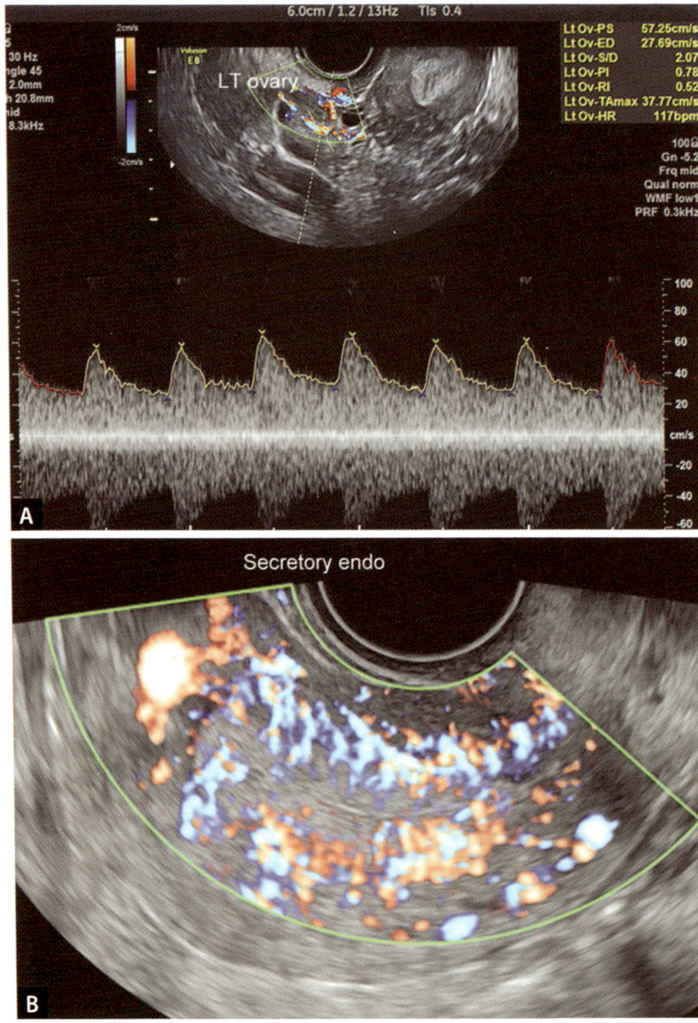

Figs. 17A and B: (A) Low-resistance blood flow of the corpus luteum demonstrated on pulse Doppler; (B) HD power Doppler showing blood flow in the secretory endometrium.

- B-mode ultrasound with Doppler is used to assess ovarian reserve and response to decide the daily dose of gonadotropins using baseline scoring.
- Pretrigger Doppler is recommended to decide precise time of trigger, type of trigger for safety and best results of IUI cycle and also to decide on how many IUI need to be done and the time of IUI.
- Luteal phase scan is important to understand the failure and do required modifications in subsequent cycles.

REFERENCES

1. Kupesic S, Kurjak A. Predictors of IVF outcome by three-dimensional ultrasound. Hum Reprod. 2002;17(4):950-5.
2. Popovic-Todorovic B, Loft A, Lindhard A, Bangsboll S, Andersson AM, Anderson AN. A prospective study of predictive factors of ovarian response in 'standard' IVF/ICSI patients treated with recombinant FSH. A suggestion for recombinant FSH dosage normogram. Hum Reprod. 2003;18(4):781-7.
3. Merce LT, Barco MJ, Bau S, Troyano JM. Prediction of ovarian response and IVF/ICSI outcome by three dimensional ultrasonography and power Doppler angiography. Eur J Obstet Gynecol Reprod Biol. 2007;132(1):93-100.

4. Ng EHU, Yeung WSB, Fong DYT, Ho PC. Effects of age on hormonal and ultrasound markers of ovarian reserve in Chinese women with proven fertility. Hum Reprod. 2003;18(10):2169-74.
5. Lam PM, Johnson IR, Rainne-Fenning NJ. Three dimensional ultrasound features of the polycystic ovary and the effect of different phenotypic expressions on these parameters. Hum Reprod. 2007;22(12):3116-23.
6. Chen MJ, Yang WS, Chen CL, Wu MY, Yang YS, Ho HN. The relationship between anti-Müllerian hormone, androgen and insulin resistance on the number of antral follicles in women with polycystic ovary syndrome. Hum Reprod. 2008;23(4):952-7.
7. Van Rooij IA, Broekmans FJM, te Velde ER, Fauser BCJM, Bancsi LFJMM, de Jong FH, et al. Serum anti-Müllerian hormone levels: a novel measure of ovarian reserve. Hum Reprod. 2002;17(12):3065-71.
8. Krishnakumar J, Agarwal A, Nambiar D, Radhakrishnan S. Comparison of antral follicle count, anti-Müllerian hormone and day 2 follicle stimulating hormone as predictor of ovarian response and clinical pregnancy rate in patient with an abnormal ovarian reserve test. Int J Reprod Contracept Obstet Gynecol. 2016;5(8):2762-7.
9. Broer SL, Mol BWJ, Hendriks D, Broekmans FJM. The role of anti-Müllerian hormone in prediction of outcome after IVF: comparison with the antral follicle count. Fertil Steril. 2009;91(3):705-14.
10. Panchal S, Nagori C. Comparison of AFC and AMH for assessment of ovarian reserve. J Hum Reprod Sci. 2012;5(3):274-8.
11. Rainne-Fenning NJ. What is in a number? The polycystic ovary revisited. Hum Reprod. 2011;26(11);3118-22.
12. Deb S, Jayaprakasan K, Campbell BK, Clewes JS, Johnson IR, Raine-Fenning NJ. Intraobserver and interobserver reliability of automated antral follicle counts made using three-dimensional ultrasound and SonoAVC. Ultrasound Obstet Gynecol. 2009;33(4):477-83.
13. Jayaprakasan K, Hopkisson J, Campbell B, Johnson I, Thornton J, Raine-Fenning N. A randomised controlled trial of 300 versus 225 IU recombinant FSH for ovarian stimulation in predicted normal responders by antral follicle count. Hum Reprod. 2007;22:1932-41.
14. te Velde ER. Advances in fertility studies and reproductive medicine. IFFS. 2007;306.
15. Lass A, Skull J, McVeigh E, Margara R, Winston RM. Measurement of ovarian volume by transvaginal sonography before ovulation induction with human menopausal gonadotrophin for in vitro fertilization can predict poor response. Hum Reprod. 1992;12(2): 294-7.
16. Zaidi J, Barber J, Kyei-Mensah A, Bekir J, Campbell S, Tan SL. Relationship of ovarian stromal blood flow at baseline ultrasound to subsequent follicular response in an in vitro fertilization program. Obstet Gynecol. 1996;88(5):779-84.
17. Engmann L, Saldkevicius P, Agrawal R, Bekir JS, Campbell S, Tan S. Value of ovarian stromal blood flow velocity measurement after pituitary suppression in the prediction of ovarian responsiveness and outcome of in vitro fertilization treatment. Fertil Steril. 1999;71(1):22-9.
18. Arora A, Gainder S, Dhaliwal L, Suri V. Clinical significance of ovarian stromal blood flow in assessment of ovarian response in stimulated cycle for in vitro fertilization. Int J Reprod Contracept Obstet Gynecol. 2015;4(5):1380-3.
19. Panchal S, Nagori C. Ultrasound-based decision making on stimulation protocol for superovulated intrauterine insemination cycles. Int J Infertil Fetal Med. 2016;7(1):7-13.
20. Jokubkeine L, Sladkevicius P, Rovas L, Valentine L. Assessment of changes in volume and vascularity of ovaries during the normal menstrual cycle using three dimensional power Doppler ultrasound. Hum Reprod. 2006;21(10):2661-8.
21. Nargund G, Doyle PE, Bourne TH, Parsons JH, Cheng WC, Campbell S, et al. Ultrasound-deviced indices of follicular blood flow before HCG administration and prediction of oocyte recovery and preimplantation embryo quality. Hum Reprod. 1996;11(11):2512-17.
22. Nargund G, Bourne TH, Doyle PE, Parsons J, Cheng W, Campbell S, et al. Association between ultrasound indices of follicular blood flow, oocyte recovery and preimplantation embryo quality. Hum Reprod. 1996;11(1): 109-13.
23. Blerkom V, Antezak M, Schrader R. The developmental potential of human oocyte is related to the dissolved oxygen content of follicular fluid: association with vascular endothelial growth factor levels and perifollicular blood flow characteristics. Hum Reprod. 1997;12(5):1047-55.
24. Panchal SY, Nagori CB. Can 3D PD be a better tool for assessing the pre HCG follicle and endometrium? A randomized study of 500 cases. Presented at 16th World Congress on

Ultrasound in Obstetrics and Gynecology, 2006, London. J Ultrasound Obstet Gynecol. 2006;28(4):504.
25. Wittmack FM, Kreger DO, Blasco L, Tureck RW, Mastroianni L Jr, Lessey BA. Effect of follicular size on oocyte retrieval, fertilization, cleavage and embryo quality in in vitro fertilization cycles: a 6 year data collection. Fertil Steril. 1994;62(6):1205-10.
26. Kyei-Mensah A, Zaidi J, Pittrof R, Shaker A, Campbell S, Tan SL. Transvaginal three-dimensional ultrasound reproducibility of ovarian and endometrial volume measurements. Fertil Steril. 1996;66(5):718-22.
27. Wu MH, Tsai SJ, Pan HA, Hsiao KY, Chang FM. Three-dimensional power Doppler imaging of ovarian stromal blood flow in women with endometriosis undergoing in vitro fertilization. Ultrasound Obstet Gynecol. 2003;21(5):480-5.
28. Vlaisavljevic V, Reljic M, Gavric Lovrec V, Zazula D, Sergent N. Measurement of perifollicular blood flow of the dominant preovulatory follicle using three dimensional power Doppler. Ultrasound Obstet Gynecol. 2003;22:520-6.
29. Merce LT. Ultrasound markers of implantation. Ultrasound Rev Obstet Gynecol. 2002;2:110-23.
30. Merce LT, Barco MJ, Kupesic S, Kurjak A. 2D and 3D power Doppler ultrasound from ovulation to implantation. In: Kurjak A, Chervenak F (Eds). Textbook of Perinatal Medicine. London: Parthenon Publishing; 2005.
31. Bourne TH, Jurkovic D, Waterstone J, Campbell S, Collins WP. Intrafollicular blood flow during human ovulation. Ultrasound Obstet Gynecol. 1991;1:53-9.
32. Hancock KL, Pereira N, Christos PJ, Petrini AC, Hughes J, Chung PH, Rosenwaks Z. Optimal lead follicle size for human chorionic gonadotropin trigger in clomiphene citrate and intrauterine insemination cycles: an analysis of 1676 treatment cycles. Fertil Steril. 2021;115(4):984-9.
33. Smith B, Porter R, Ahuja K, Craft I. Ultrasonic assessment of endometrial changes in stimulated cycles in an in vitro fertilization and embryo transfer program. J In Vitro Fertil Embryo Transf. 1984;1:233-8.
34. Applebaum M. The 'steel' or 'teflon' endometrium—ultrasound visualization of endometrial vascularity in IVF patients and outcome. Presented at the third World Congress of Ultrasound in Obstetrics and Gynaecology. Ultrasound Obstet Gynecol. 1993;3(Suppl 2):10.
35. Yang JH, Wu MY, Chen CD, Jiang MC, Ho HN, Yang YS. Association of endometrial blood flow as determined by a modified color Doppler technique with subsequent outcome of in-vitro fertilization. Hum Reprod. 1999;14:1606-10.
36. Chein LW, Au HK, Chen PL, Xiao J, Tzeng CR. Assessment of uterine receptivity by the endometrial-subendometrial blood flow distribution pattern in women undergoing in vitro fertilization-embryo transfer. Fertil Steril. 2002;78(2):245-51.
37. Nagori C, Panchal S. Endometrial vascularity: its relation to implantation rates. Int J Infert Fetal Med. 2012;3(2):48-50.
38. Zaidi J, Campbell S, Pittrof R, Tan SL. Endometrial thickness, morphology, vascular penetration and velocimetry in predicting implantation in an in vitro fertilization program. Ultrasound Obstet Gynecol. 1995;6(3):191-8.
39. Steer CV, Campbell S, Tan SL, Crayford T, Mills C, Mason BA, et al. The use of transvaginal colour flow imaging after in vitro fertilization to identify optimum uterine conditions before embryo transfer. Fertil Steril. 1992;57(2):372-6.
40. Zaidi J, Pittrof R, Shaker A, Kyei-Mensah A, Campbell S, Tan SL. Assessment of uterine artery blood flow on the day of human chorionic gonadotrophin administration by transvaginal colour Doppler ultrasound in an in vitro fertilization program. Fertil Steril. 1996;65:377-81.
41. Coulam CB, Stern JJ, Soenksen DM, Britten S, Bustillo M. Comparison of pulsatility indexes on the day of oocyte retrieval and embryo transfer. Hum Reprod. 1995;10:82-4.
42. Cacciatore B, Simberg N, Fusaro P, Tiitinen A. Transvaginal Doppler study of uterine artery blood flow in in vitro fertilization embryo transfer cycles. Fertil Steril. 1996;66:130-4.
43. Raga F, Bonilla-Musoles F, Casan EM, Klein O, Bonilla F. Assessment of endometrial volume by three-dimensional ultrasound prior to embryo transfer: clues to endometrial receptivity. Hum Reprod. 1999;14:2851-4.
44. Kupesic S, Bekavac I, Bjelos D, Kurjak A. Assessment of endometrial receptivity by transvaginal colour Doppler and three-dimensional power Doppler ultrasonography in patients undergoing in vitro fertilization procedures. J Ultrasound Med. 2001;20:125-34.
45. Kupesić S, Kurjak A, Vujisić S, Petrović Z. Luteal phase defect: comparison between Doppler velocimetry, histological and hormonal markers. Ultrasound Obstet Gynecol. 1997;9(2):105-12.
46. Glock JL, Brumsted JR. Colour flow pulsed Doppler ultrasound in diagnosing luteal phase defect. Fertil Steril. 1995;64:500-4.

CHAPTER 5

Stimulation Protocol for Intrauterine Insemination

INTRODUCTION

Ovarian stimulation is the main pillar for success of intrauterine insemination (IUI) treatment. There are multiple advantages of superovulation or controlled ovarian stimulation. The goal is to develop 2–3 follicles.

Advantages of controlled ovarian hyperstimulation (COH):

- It increases the number of oocytes for fertilization so there is more chance of fertilization.[1]
- It increases ovarian steroids that improve chances of fertilization and implantation.
- Subtle hormonal deficiencies are corrected.
- Luteal phase defect is corrected.
- Increases implantation window as several oocytes are released over protracted period.
- Ovulation induction and IUI both independently increase pregnancy rates. A meta-analysis by Guzik et al. have shown that combination improves pregnancy rate.[2,3]

Relative effectiveness of clomiphene citrate, letrozole, or gonadotropins for ovulation induction in IUI-with ovarian stimulation cycles in terms of cumulative live birth rate, further studies are suggested by some authors.[4]

STIMULATION PROTOCOL

No Stimulation

Pregnancy rate varies from 2 to 8% in a nonstimulated cycle. It is always lower than stimulated cycles, as in stimulated cycles, more follicles develop but also has higher multiple pregnancy rate and risk of ovarian hyperstimulation syndrome (OHSS). Many centers, including Bourne Hall clinic, London, offer natural cycle IUI. But in India, natural cycle IUI is never preferred because of its low pregnancy rate.

Clomiphene Citrate for Superovulation

Clomiphene is given in a dose of 50–100 mg from Day 5–9. Clomiphene has not given higher pregnancy rate, as cycle fecundability in spontaneous and clomiphene citrate (CC)-induced cycle is the same (6–13%) as compared to gonadotropins (14–24%).[2] Lower pregnancy rate with CC in IUI cycles is because of adverse effect of CC on endometrium.[5] Ovarian stimulation with letrozole may significantly increase live birth rates controlling multiple pregnancy rates compared to CC and only human menopausal gonadotropin (HMG).[6] For all our IUIs, we use gonadotropins, which give higher pregnancy rate.

One of the uses of CC is to prevent the luteinizing hormone (LH) surge. We can start the stimulation with gonadotropin and after 10-mm size of the follicle, clomiphene is added to prevent premature LH surge. LH surge is suppressed but it does not increase the pregnancy rate.[7] For better success of IUI, always give gonadotropins alone. Because you are going to try 3–6 cycles of IUI before in vitro fertilization (IVF), IUI must be done with gonadotropins. Treatment with gonadotropins seems to be more effective. On the basis of current data, IVF or ICSI is not more effective than IUI with gonadotropins.[8] The same conclusion was also derived by Tjon RT et al. for unexplained male infertility.[9]

Gonadotropins

Gonadotropins with IUI have higher pregnancy rate than CC or natural intercourse. It has 10–15% chance of pregnancy per cycle as compared to 1–2% with natural cycle in unexplained infertility. A meta-analysis clearly shows gonadotropins to be more effective than CC.[10] Different types of gonadotropins are available but meta-analysis of different gonadotropins did not show one to be superior over other.[10] Even by increasing the dose, it does not improve the pregnancy rate, though it increases multiple pregnancy rate.[11] Low dose HMG with IUI has given higher pregnancy rate than CC with IUI and is more cost-effective. But in our experience, FSH (follicle-stimulating hormone) gives much better results in IUI cycles than HMG.

Protocols for Gonadotropins

The dose of gonadotropin is decided according to the baseline scan. Baseline scan decides whether it is normal ovary, polycystic ovary syndrome (PCOS), or poor responding ovary. This aspect is discussed in the Chapter 4 of this book. The baseline score[12] to decide the required dose of gonadotropins is very useful to prevent OHSS and also to reduce cycle cancellations.

- *Conventional protocol* ***(Fig. 1)***: Follicle-stimulating hormone is started from Day 5 of the cycle in a dose of 75 IU per day for 5 days after confirming on transvaginal scan that all follicles are smaller than 10 mm in diameter. For all practical purposes, gonadotropins are always started from Day 5 in IUI cycles and from Day 2 in IVF cycles. The rationale is that

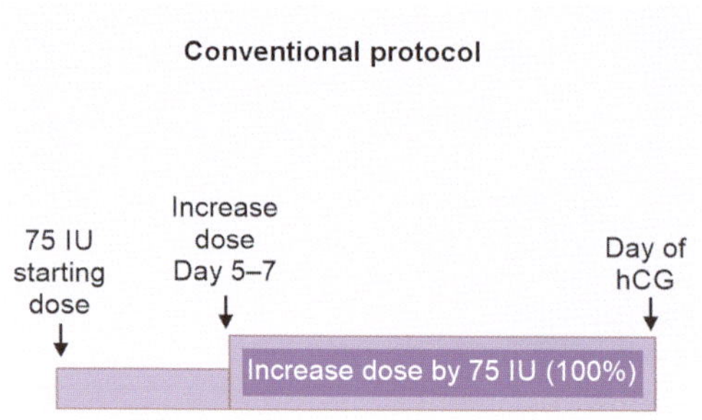

Fig. 1: Diagrammatic presentation of conventional protocol. (hCG: human chorionic gonadotropin)

  by Day 5, the follicle dominance is already established and after that when FSH is started, it results in mono- or bifollicular development only. After five injections, the patient is called on Day 10 of the cycle for scan, if on the day on which gonadotropin is started, all follicles were <10 mm. On Day 10, if the endometrium is growing or follicle is growing beyond 10 mm, continue the same dose till the day of human chorionic gonadotropin (hCG), otherwise increase the dose to 150 IU for 3 days, i.e., on Day 10, 11, and 12. In majority of patients, follicular growth occurs. If follicle does not grow beyond 10 mm, it is a poor responding ovary and the diagnosis of normal responding ovary was not correct. In this case, dose may have to be increased to 225 IU daily and follicular growth will be seen. Once follicular growth is documented, same dose is continued.[13]
- *Step-down protocol* ***(Fig. 2)***: This protocol is especially for poor responding ovary. Stimulation is started with 150–225 IU daily dose from Day 5–9 till a follicle grows to 10 mm. Then one can decrease the dose till follicle grows to 14 mm and then further decreased and continued till follicle attains maturity. This protocol mimics the FSH levels similar to what is normally present in our body and gives 1–2 follicles.

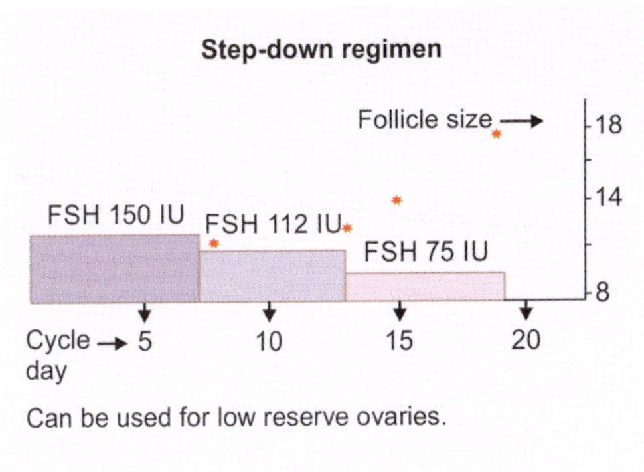

Fig. 2: Diagrammatic presentation of step-down protocol. (FSH: follicle-stimulating hormone)

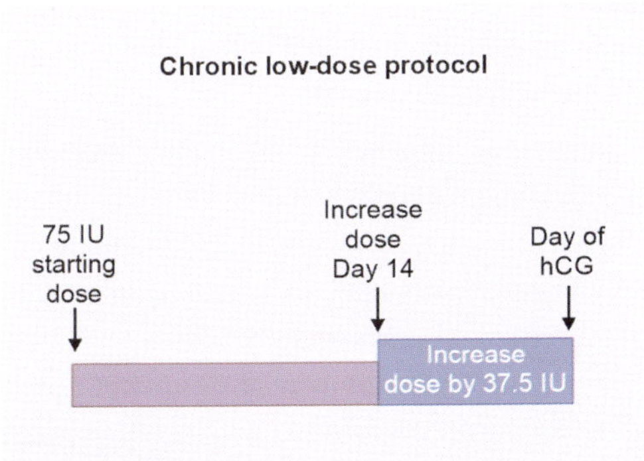

Fig. 3: Diagrammatic presentation of chronic low-dose protocol. (hCG: human chorionic gonadotropin)

- *Chronic low-dose protocol* **(Fig. 3)**: This protocol is for high-responding patients; starting dose can be calculated from the table of baseline score[12] (refer to Chapter 4) and accordingly 37.5 or 75 IU of FSH is started from Day 5. The same dose is continued for 14 days. In-between, once or twice ultrasound should be done to check for development of follicle. If the follicle during this period grows to 10–12 mm, continue the same dose till follicle grows to maturity. If the follicle growth is not documented, then even do not increase the dose till 14 complete days of stimulation. If no follicle growth beyond 10 mm even after 14 days, then the dose is increased by 50% of the starting dose. That means if the starting dose was 75 IU, the dose is increased by 37.5 IU and is made 112.5 IU and this dose is given for 7 days. In majority of cases, the follicle grows. But, if it does not, then in rare cases, further dose may be increased after 7 days. In these cases, especially recombinant FSH is considered better as it allows precise dose titration.

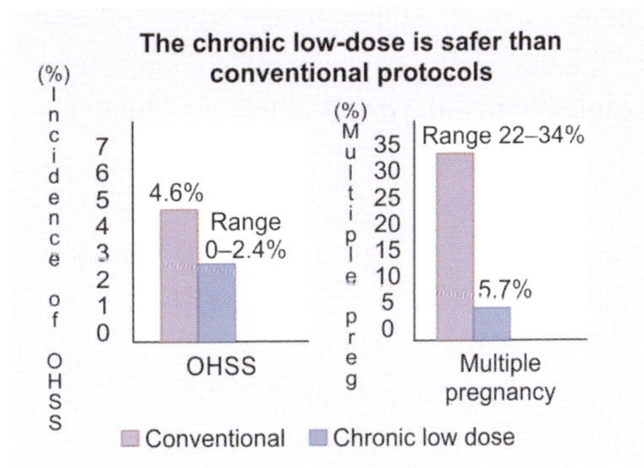

Fig. 4: Graphic diagram showing less ovarian hyperstimulation syndrome (OHSS) and lesser multiple pregnancy rates with chronic low-dose protocol.

Advantages of chronic low-dose protocol are[12,14] ***(Fig. 4)****:*

- Monofollicular development
- Multiple pregnancies can be avoided.
- Premature LH surge is avoided.
- Antagonists are not required.
- Implantation rate is improved.

Recent Cochrane review, 2007 shows gonadotropin is most effective drug when IUI is combined with controlled ovarian hyperstimulation (COH).[15]

Clomiphene Citrate + Gonadotropin

Clomiphene is often combined with gonadotropins with the idea that it would decrease the requirement of gonadotropins. Clomiphene citrate by its direct effect on ovary increases the sensitivity of ovary to gonadotropins. This combination, therefore, has higher risk of ovarian hyperstimulation and multiple pregnancies. Increased LH secretion induced by CC may reduce the likelihood of conception.[16] CC increases LH levels that are detrimental to ova and by adding HMG, further LH is added. LH may reach ceiling level and destroy the quality of the ovum. The poor pregnancy rate with clomiphene citrate is because of high LH, which will remain in spite of adding gonadotropins. Pregnancy rate with CC + human menopausal gonadotrophin (HMG) is same as for CC alone.[17] Therefore, in our opinion, CC + HMG should never be used for IUI cycles or for regular treatment.

This does not occur if only FSH is given for ovulation induction. Instead, letrozole is a better drug to be combined with gonadotropins. This will be discussed later.

Low-dose FSH protocol is recommended by Professor Roy Homburg as a first line of treatment for ovulation induction instead of CC. The study has shown to double the pregnancy rates, with reduced treatment pregnancy interval and more singleton pregnancies.[18] Some workers have tried giving gonadotropins on alternate days or every 3rd day. But this is not recommended. Gonadotropins should be always given daily to get good results.

In the 'PROTRIALS' study, fixed dose of FSH 75 IU had a lower response in 2/3rd of the patients. Age, BMI and FSH predicted hyper-response well. There was no clear correlation between serum AMH and ovarian response. Individualizing dose thus can prevent hyper-response.[19]

Letrozole + Gonadotropins

When letrozole is given from Day 3–7, it develops follicle. Estradiol is secreted from the follicle; this is sensed by hypothalamus and reduces FSH and LH. Now, if FSH is added, this follicle gets a boost to grow. Moreover, as LH decreases, ovum quality is not spoilt, as it may occur when CC was used instead of letrozole. As letrozole raises androgen, it sensitizes follicle to FSH and so lower dose of FSH is required. Therefore, letrozole + gonadotropin gives same pregnancy rates as gonadotropin alone stimulation with lesser dose of FSH (lower cost). In poor responders also, we get endogenous FSH by giving letrozole and exogenous FSH is given, so lower dose of FSH is required. We routinely use this stimulation protocol for superovulation in IUI.[20-22] Peeraer K et al. showed that low dose gonadotropin stimulation is cost-effective and gives better pregnancy rate than CC, when combined with IUI.[11]

Baseline Scan and Deciding the Stimulation Protocol

This scan is done when hormonal levels are at baseline on Day 2-3 of the menstrual cycle. The ovaries are silent and have no active follicle or corpus luteum at this stage. Route of scan has to be transvaginal always to allow better resolution and more anatomical details of ovary and endometrium. All the scans are done using B mode ultrasound with color Doppler, pulse Doppler, 3D ultrasound and 3D power Doppler. Using color Doppler in this assessment is mandatory because a large number of biochemical or hormonal changes occur during the menstrual cycle, which reflect as vascular and morphological changes in the ovaries and uterus and vascular changes can be assessed by Doppler.

We have devised a baseline scoring system for individualizing the dose of FSH, based on age, BMI, antral follicle count, ovarian volume, ovarian stromal resistance index (RI) and peak systolic velocity (PSV).

Precise calculation of antral follicle count therefore can help in predicting the ovarian response. This can be done on 2D ultrasound or by 3D with inversion mode rendering and Sono AVC a specialized 3D ultrasound software for calculation of antral follicle number and volumes. This method is more precise as there is least chance of follicles being missed or being counted twice because of color coding. But post-processing is required for accurate calculations. It takes longer to perform, because of the need for post-processing, and obtains values that are lower than those obtained by the 2D and 3D-MPV techniques.[23,24]

AFC and ovarian volume provide direct measurements of ovarian reserve.[25]

This may be calculated on 2D ultrasound by measuring three longest orthogonal diameters and using x x y x z x 0.523 cm or on 3D ultrasound by VOCAL software. Inclusion of stromal blood flows as one of the decision-making parameters is also considered. It has been shown that measurement of ovarian stromal flow in early follicular phase is related to subsequent ovarian response in IVF treatment.[26]

Based on all these facts and findings, it is understood that ovaries that have high resistance, low velocity flow require higher doses of gonadotrophins for stimulation. Whereas those with low resistance, high velocity flow requires lower doses of gonadotropins for stimulation.

Score	***1***	***2***	***3***	***4***	***5***
Age	>40	35.1–40	30.1–35	25.1–30	<25
BMI	>30	30–28.1	28–25.1	25–22.1	<22
AFC	<5	5–10	10–15	15–20	>20
Ov volume	<3	3.1–5	5.1–7	7.1–10	>10
Stromal RI	>0.75	0.75–0.66	0.65–0.56	0.55–0.45	<0.45
Stromal PSV	<3	3.1–5	5.1–7	7.1–10	>10

The ovulation induction in all patients was done by rFSH and the stimulation doses were based on the scores of individual patient based on the above-mentioned table. The doses according to the patient's score were decided as follows:

≥25	25 IU
20–24	37.5 IU
15–20	75 IU
10–15	112.5 IU
6–10	150 IU

Dose alteration if required is done as following algorithm.

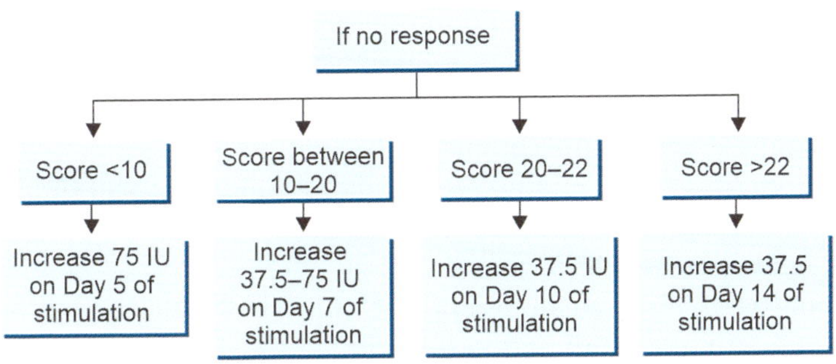

As per the results of our study, the scoring system devised in this study for deciding the stimulation protocol is highly reliable for safe planning of stimulation protocols in ART cycles as the OHSS rates and cycle cancellation rates due to poor response are negligible. Multiple pregnancy rates are also acceptable. This study we believe may prove to be an important guide for safe use of gonadotropins for ovulation induction in ART cycles.[27]

ROLE OF AGONIST

Gonadotropin-releasing hormone (GnRH) agonist is not used routinely in IUI protocols. It increases the total dose of gonadotropins consumed and increases incidence of OHSS and multiple pregnancy rates. It has no advantage in IUI protocols and we never use these for IUI cycles.

Instead, GnRH antagonists may be used in IUI protocols.

ROLE OF GnRH ANTAGONIST

In about 24% of IUI cycles, premature LH surge is documented. Adding GnRH antagonist in cycles with mild ovarian hyperstimulation in an IUI program does not increase live birth rate.[7] Though, it is very useful in thin lean PCOS patients in whom LH is tonically high. Here, antagonist is given when follicle size of 14 mm is reached till the day of trigger. It prevents premature LH surge and improves the quality of ova and embryo, which in turn gives higher pregnancy rates.[5] Use of GnRH antagonist with COH (controlled ovarian hyperstimulation) and IUI significantly increases pregnancy rates and reduces the incidence of premature luteinization. It allows more follicles to grow to more than 18-mm diameter and improves pregnancy rates.[28] But, routine use of antagonist is not recommended by other studies and it does not increase the pregnancy rate.[10] In patients with no premature LH surge or non-PCOS, it does not increase the pregnancy rate. So, antagonist cannot be given to all patients in IUI.[7] Antagonist helps in multifollicular development and increases pregnancy rate in older people and in these cases, multiple pregnancy rarely occurs. So, it is used when women are >28 years.[29]

Which gonadotropin to be used?

There is a lot of confusion about this, as there are several brands available for gonadotropins and each one claims a particular product to be the best. Gonadotropins are made from menopausal urine and are known as urinary gonadotropins, or these may be recombinant products. To understand why later is considered to be better, let us first understand physiology related to FSH. FSH that is secreted after menstruation is least bioactive and is more in amount. While FSH that is secreted during preovulatory period has highest bioactivity and is little in amount. The bioactivity of FSH also decreases significantly close to menopause and is very low after menopause. Recombinant FSH (r-FSH) is prepared from Chinese larva and is cloned in such a way that it mimics preovulatory FSH having highest bioactivity. Whereas, urinary FSH is produced from menopausal urine and, therefore, has the least bioactivity. The potency of urinary FSH is much less than recombinant FSH. Recombinant FSH has a bioactivity of 10,000 IU, while highly purified (HP) FSH has bioactivity of 9,000 IU and other gonadotropins have much less bioactivity **(Table 1)**.

TABLE 1: Type of gonadotropin and its specific bioactivity.

Product	*Specific bioactivity*
HMG (1950)	8 IU/mg protein
uFSH (1980)	100–150 IU/mg protein
uHMG-HP	2,000 IU/mg protein
uFSH-HP (1990)	9,000 IU/mg protein
rFSH (1995)	10,000 IU/mg protein

(FSH: follicle-stimulating hormone; HMG: human menopausal gonadotropin)

So, we use rFSH or at the most FSH-HP. Clinically, we have observed that 75 IU rFSH is equivalent to 150 units of urinary FSH. That means dose of rFSH can be 50% less than that of urinary products. So, accordingly dose should be adjusted.[30]

Second question is whether FSH or HMG should be used?

In IUI, downregulation with agonist is not done. So, endogenous LH is always present and is in normal range. So, exogenous LH is not required. If HMG is used in this case, LH accumulates in late follicular phase and may cross the ceiling level. So, it may spoil the quality of the ova and so FSH is always preferred than HMG. Moreover, in all PCOS patients, LH is on the higher side and HMG will further increase in LH level, which is detrimental to ova. Therefore, in IUI, FSH is preferred to HMG.

Human menopausal gonadotropin may be required on patients of >35 years of age and has not given good response in spite of normal AFC or AMH. These are the patients in whom ovarian stromal flow is low because of low LH or LH polymorphism may be present. These are the only few cases in whom LH supplementation may be required and HMG stimulation may be used.

CARRY HOME MESSAGE

- Intrauterine insemination (IUI) without stimulation has poor pregnancy rate.
- Gonadotropin stimulation has higher pregnancy rate.
- Dosage should be according to baseline scan.
- Letrozole with gonadotropins is a very effective protocol.
- Recombinant FSH requires lower dosage.
- Antagonist is useful in PCOS patients.

REFERENCES

1. Van Rumste MM, Custers IM, Van der Veen F, Van Wely M, Evers JL, Mol BW. The influence of number of follicles on pregnancy rate in intrauterine insemination with ovarian stimulation: a meta-analysis. Hum Reprod Update. 2008;14(6):563-70.
2. Guzick DS, Sullivan MW, Adamson GD, Cedars MI, Falk RJ, Peterson EP, et al. Efficacy of treatment for unexplained infertility. Fertil Steril. 1998;70(2):S90-6.
3. Verhulst SM, Cohlens BJ, Hughes E, te Velde E, Heineman MJ. Intrauterine insemination for unexplained subfertility. Cochrane Database Syst Rev. 2006;(4):CD001838.
4. van Eekelen R, Wang R, Danhof NA, Mol F, Mochtar M, Mol BW, van Wely M. Cost-effectiveness of ovarian stimulation agents for IUI in couples with unexplained subfertility. Hum Reprod. 2021;36(5):1288-95.
5. Biljan MM, Mahutte NG, Tulandi T, Tan SL. Prospective double blind trial of the correlation between time of administration and antioestrogenic effects of clomiphene citrate in reproductive end organs. Fertil Steril. 1999;71(4):633-8.
6. Huang S, Wang R, Rong Li, Wang H, Qiao J, Mol BW. Ovarian stimulation in infertile women treated with the use of intrauterine insemination: a cohort study from China. Fertil Steril. 2018;109(5):872-8.
7. Cantineau AEP, Cohlen BJ, Klip H, Heineman MJ, Dutch IUI study Group Collaborators. The addition of GnRH antagonists in intrauterine insemination cycles with mild ovarian hyperstimulation does not increase live birth rates: a randomized, double-blinded, placebo-controlled trial. Hum Reprod. 2011; 26(5):1104-11.
8. Crown DD, Bates GW. Evidence based approach to unexplained infertility: a systematic review. Fertil Steril. 2016;105(6):1566-74.
9. Tjon-Kun-Pat RI, Tajik P, Zafarmand MH, Bensdorp AJ, Bossuyt PMM, Oosterhuis GJE, et al. IUI or IVF as first line treatment in unexplained subfertility: the conundrum of treatment selection markers. Hum Reprod. 2017;32(5):1028-32.
10. Cantineau AE, Cohlen BJ, Heineman MJ. Ovarian stimulation protocols (anti-oestrogens, gonadotrophins with subfertility. Cochrane Database Syst Rev. 2007;(2):CD005356.
11. Peeraer K, Debrock S, De Loecker P, Tomassetti C, Laenen A, Welkenhuysen M, et al. Low dose HMG v/s CC in subfertile couples

treated with IUI: a randomized controlled trial. Hum Reprod. 2015;30(5):1079-88.
12. Panchal S, Nagori CB. Ultrasound based decision making on stimulation protocols for superovulated IUI cycles. IJIFM. 2016;7(1):7-13.
13. Homburg R, Insler V. Ovulation induction in perspective. Hum Reprod Update. 2002;8(5):449-62.
14. Dale O, Tanbo T, Lunde O, Abyholm T. Ovulation induction with low dose follicle stimulating hormone in women with polycystic ovarian syndrome. Acta Obstet Gynecol Scand. 1993;72(1):43-6.
15. Cohlen BJ, Heineman MJ. Ovarian stimulation protocols (anti-oestrogens, gonadotrophins with and without GnRH agonist/antagonist). Cochrane Database Syst Rev. 2007;(2):CD005356.
16. Hamilton-Fairley D, Franks S. Common problems in induction of ovulation. Baillieres Clin Obstet Gynaecol. 1990;4:609-25.
17. Vargyas JM, Moernte C, Shangold G, Marrs RP. The effect of different methods of ovarian stimulation for human in vitro fertilization and embryo replacement. Fertil Steril. 1984; 42(5):745-9.
18. Homburg R, Hendriks L, Konig TE, Anderson RA, Balen AH, Brincat M, et al. Clomiphene citrate or low dose FSH for the first line treatment of infertile women with anovulation associated with polycystic ovary syndrome: a prospective randomized multinational study. Hum Reprod. 2012;27(2):468-73.
19. Rutten A, van Ballegooijen H, Broekmans F, Cohlen B, et al. Insights into ovarian response with a fixed low dose FSH stimulation in an IUI programme: the PROTRIALS study. Hum Reprod. 2022;37(7):1440-50.
20. Garcia-Valesco JA. The use of aromatase inhibitors in invitro fertilization. Fertil Steril. 2012;98(6):1356-8.
21. Mitwally MFM, Casper RF. Aromatase inhibition reduces gonadotrophin dose required for controlled ovarian stimulation in women with unexplained infertility. Hum Reprod. 2003;18(8):1588-97.
22. Badawy MA, Sorky M, Mousa N, Claessens A, Esfandiari N, Gotleib L, et al. Letrazole co-treatment in infertile women of 40 years old and older receiving controlled ovarian stimulation and IUI. Fertil Steril. 2009;91(6):2501-7.
23. Rainne-Fenning NJ. What is in a number? The polycystic ovary revisited. Hum Reprod. 2011;26(11);3118-22.
24. Deb, S, Jayaprakasan, K, Campbell B. K, Clewes, J. S, Johnson IR, Raine-Fenning N. J. Ultrasound in Obstetrics and Gynecology, Volume 33, Number 4, April 2009 , pp. 477-483(7).
25. ER te Velde,et al, Advances in fertility studies and reproductive medicine. IFFS. 2007; 306.
26. Zaidi J, Barber J, Kyei-Mensah A et al. Relationship of ovarian stromal blood flow at baseline ultrasound to subsequent follicular response in an in vitro fertilization program. Obstet Gynecol. 1996; 88:779-84.
27. Panchal S, Nagori CB. Ultrasound based decision making on stimulation protocol for superovulated IUI cycles. IJIFM. 2016, 7(1): 7-13.
28. Bakas P, Konidaris S, Liapis A, Gregoriou O, Tzanakaki D, Creatsas G. Role of gonado-trophin-releasing hormone antagonist in the management of subfertile couples with IUI and COS. Fertil Steril. 2011;95(6):2024-8.
29. Monraisin O, Chancel-Debordeaux L, Chiron A, Floret S, Cens S, Bourrinet S, et al. Evaluation of intrauterine insemination practices: A one year prospective study in seven French assisted reproduction centers. Fertil Steril. 2016;105(6):1589-93.
30. Mattoras R, Osma C, Exposito A, Crisol L, Pijoan JI. rFSH versus highly purified FSH in IUI: systematic review and meta-analysis. Fertil Steril. 2011;95(6):1937-42.

CHAPTER

6

Ovulation Trigger

INTRODUCTION

Ovulation trigger is the most important step in success of intrauterine insemination (IUI). The timing of trigger wins half the battle. Ovulation trigger, i.e., surrogate luteinizing hormone (LH) surge, with human chorionic gonadotropin (hCG) is routinely given to majority of patients. Ovulation trigger is required to time ovulation, especially if procedures such as IUI or ovum pick-up are to be done because basal body temperature chart (BBT chart) or urinary LH kits cannot exactly tell when the ovulation will occur. Ovum survives for 6–8 hours after ovulation and so if IUI is not timed correctly, pregnancy rate will be very low.

What does the LH surge or trigger do?

- It induces mucinification of cumulus oophorus allowing oocyte to release.
- It provokes resumption of meiosis that is arrested at prophase of first meiotic division and is converted to metaphase II.
- It triggers follicular rupture.
- It stimulates cytokines for implantation.

Characteristics of LH surge:

- LH surge lasts for 40–50 hours.
- It has ascending phase of 14 hours, peak plateau for 14 hours, and descending phase for 20 hours, i.e., total 48 hours.[1]
- LH level increases by 10–20 times higher.
- This is because of positive feedback of estrogen when it is 150 pg/mL per follicle.
- Ovulation occurs after 36 hours of onset of LH surge.
- Meiosis starts after 14–18 hours of onset of LH surge.
- Level of LH 100 IU/mL and FSH 25–30 IU/mL is considered normal.

DRUGS FOR OVULATION TRIGGER

- Human chorionic gonadotropin (hCG)
- Gonadotrophin-releasing hormone agonist (GnRHa)

Human Chorionic Gonadotropin

Characteristics

- It has two to four times more binding affinity than LH.
- It has a biological half-life of more than 24 hours as compared 60 minutes for endogenous LH. This is so because beta-subunit of hCG is highly glycosylated and has a longer half-life.
- It stimulates the secretion of vascular endothelial growth factor (VEGF), which causes ovarian hyperstimulation syndrome (OHSS).
- Subcutaneous or intramuscular routes have same serum levels and same pregnancy rates.[2]
- Human chorionic gonadotropin is used for ovulation trigger since about 30 years.
- It activates the same receptors as that of LH on corpus luteum.
- Bioavailability is less in obese women after giving hCG and so for obese women 10,000 IU is the standard dose for trigger instead of 5,000 IU.

- No difference in oocyte yield is found with 5,000 IU or 10,000 IU of hCG.[3]
- Delayed hCG administration in agonist or antagonist cycle gives poor pregnancy rate according to some studies but others have similar results.
- Human chorionic gonadotropin trigger is given in WHO group-1 patients.
- When hCG is used, its effect lasts for 5 days to maintain corpus luteum. So, luteal phase deficiency (LPD) is not common in initial days in hCG trigger.
- Mitwally et al. also reported that hCG administration is associated with favorable outcome in ovulation induction.[4]

Side Effects

- It causes multiple follicles to rupture because of its sustained luteotropic effect. So, there is high level of E2 and P, which is detrimental for implantation.
- Multiple follicles rupture and give multiple pregnancy.
- Human chorionic gonadotropin triggers more follicles and gives high E2 and progesterone that decrease endogenous LH causing LPD after 5 days.[5,6]
- It stimulates VEGF, which is direct cause of OHSS when there are multiple follicles.[7] Whenever E2 is >1,600 pg/mL, hCG should not be given. Instead, GnRHa should be given as a trigger. One may do only ultrasound instead of assessing E2 level and can predict OHSS by ovarian volume. This is discussed in the Chapter 4. Do not give hCG when OHSS is likely.

Recombinant hCG

Its structure, absorption pattern, distribution, and metabolism are similar to hCG. It is a pure form and theoretically safe. Its maximum concentration is reached in 12–24 hours and biological half-life is 38 hours. Its efficacy and safety is similar to uhCG.[8] The dose is 250 µg that has the same bioactivity as that of 6,500 IU of uhCG. Recombinant hCG has no allergic reaction and there is no failure of ovulation. It has ease of use for patients and improved efficacy for ovulation and luteal phase support.

Gonadotropin-releasing Hormone Agonist

Characteristics

- It produces LH surge as efficiently as hCG for oocyte maturation and this was first suggested by Itskovitz in 1988.[9]
- It produces FSH surge also with LH surge, in contrast to hCG, but its role has not been established in humans. It has already been established in rats.[10]
- Both the surges are higher than with hCG used as trigger.
- There is no difference in oocyte maturation and ovulation.
- LH surge due to GnRHa is 24–36 hours as compared to natural surge, which is 48 hours in length, and hCG surge is for 6 days.
- It has only two phases. It has a short ascending limb of >4 hours and long descending limb of >20 hours.[11]
- The initial rise is because of flare-up. It leads to LH surge, which is of high peak value and shorter duration than natural LH and hCG.
- Multiple doses do not prolong surge.
- It can induce LH surge in antagonist cycle indicating that pituitary response to GnRHa and is preserved even in antagonist cycle.[12]
- Vascular endothelial growth factor and other substances such as angiopoietin-2 (destabilizing factor) are significantly decreased in follicular fluid after GnRHa trigger. This plays major role in decreasing OHSS.[13]
- GnRHa trigger increases antiestrogenic factors and helps in decreasing the risk of OHSS.

Advantages

- Estradiol and progesterone levels are lower, which can be managed by replacement.
- Instead, if the levels are supraphysiological, these are detrimental for implantation.[5,6]
- Short duration of surge of 24–36 hours is more physiological and only few follicles are converted into corpus luteum.[14]
- It reduces the risk of OHSS because of complete luteolysis[15] and decreased expression of VEGF.
- Pituitary response to GnRHa is preserved even in antagonist cycle. OHSS-free clinic concept uses antagonist to prevent premature LH surge with agonist trigger.[16]
- Here, GnRHa replaces antagonist and gives flare-up effect and releases FSH and LH from pituitary for triggering ovulation.
- It causes FSH surge, which promotes formation of LH receptors in luteinizing granulosa cells, nuclear maturation, and cumulus expansion.[17] It is useful to prevent luteinized unruptured follicle (LUF).

Disadvantages

- When GnRHa trigger is given, advantage of initial flare-up of FSH and LH is taken but the duration is very short. This can complete meiosis and may rupture the follicle but cannot support the luteal phase.
- If LH is suppressed in the previous cycles because of OC pills, it may give poor response and LH surge may be low.
- Dual trigger with 1,000–1,500 units of hCG has given good results in IVF (in vitro fertilization), but it is not tested in IUI.
- High total doses of gonadotropin also suppress endogenous LH and so GnRHa may give poor response for the LH surge.
- Patients with higher BMI, i.e., obese patients, or lower BMI <22 kg/m^2, i.e., thin lean polycystic ovary syndrome (PCOS), may give poor response.

Contraindications of GnRHa

- Hypothalamic dysfunction
- Oral contraceptive pills taken for a long duration or GnRHA depot taken for downregulation. In such patients, if GnRHa is given as a trigger in treatment cycle, it gives poor response.[18]
- Hypogonadotropic hypogonadism

Indications of GnRHa Trigger in IUI

- In PCOS when there is multifollicular development, GnRHa should be given as a trigger instead of hCG. IUI should be done at 36–38 hours as is done with hCG trigger. Ideally, in PCOS patients, chronic low-dose protocol is chosen as discussed in Chapter 5 and with this, multiple follicles will not develop. But, to avoid OHSS, whenever there is multifollicular growth, GnRHa trigger is given. With judicious luteal support, pregnancy rates are very good. We have never converted IUI cycle to IVF.
- In patients with LUF with hCG, GnRHa may be an effective trigger, as it also gives FSH surge, which may help in rupture of the follicle, e.g., in endometriosis.

Luteal Support in GnRHa Trigger in IUI

- Vaginal progesterone 400 mg BD and estradiol valerate 2 mg BD should be given.
- Subcutaneous injection of aqueous progesterone 25 mg daily along with estradiol valerate 4 mg can be given.
- 1,500 IU of hCG at the time of IUI can rescue the corpus luteum and estrogen and progesterone can be given as mentioned earlier.[19]
- 1,000 IU of hCG along with GnRHa trigger can also work as a good luteal support with estrogen and progesterone.

Dosage

Various dosage schedules are described in literature:

- 500–1,000 μg of leuprolide acetate
- Two injections of 500–1,000 μg leuprolide acetate 12 hour apart
- Two injections of 0.1 mg of decapeptyl at a time
- Intranasal Buserelin 50–200 pg or Triptorelin 0.2 mg
- 2,000 μg leuprolide acetate stat

Unfortunately, which compound, what dose, and when to give are still not standardized.

When 5,000 IU of hCG and 0.2 mg of decapeptyl were given, pregnancy rates were 36% as compared to 22% when only hCG was given. So, dual trigger may be used routinely for better results.

When to give trigger?

This has been discussed in detail in the Chapter 4. I will like to emphasize here that we use only ultrasound for monitoring with no hormonal investigations to decide the time of trigger.

CARRY HOME MESSAGE

- Luteinizing hormone surge is mandatory for ovulation.
- Follicle-stimulating hormone surge is useful, but its role is not understood.
- Human chorionic gonadotropin surge is required in controlled ovarian hyperstimulation (COH) and IUI cycles.
- Human chorionic gonadotropin surge does not require luteal support in initial phase, i.e., for 5 days.
- Gonadotropin-releasing hormone agonist, as ovulation trigger avoids OHSS.
- It causes LPD that requires judicious luteal support.
- 1,500 IU of hCG can rescue corpus luteum in agonist trigger when given at the time of pick up or IUI.
- Recombinant LH for trigger is very costly.
- Dual trigger with agonist and hCG is beneficial.

REFERENCES

1. Hoff JD, Quigley ME, Yen SSC. Hormonal dynamics at midcycle: a re-evaluation. J Clin Endocrinal Metab. 1983;57(4):792-6.
2. Elkind-Hirsch KE, Bello S, Esparcia L, Phillips K, Sheiko A, McNichol M, et al. Serum human gonadotropin levels are correlated with body mass index rather than route of administration in women undergoing in vitro fertilization-embryo transfer using human menopausal gonadotropin and intracytoplasmic sperm injection. Fertil Steril. 2001;75(4):700-4.
3. Shaltout AM, Eid MS, Shohayeb AA. Does triggering ovulation by 5000 IU of hCG affect ICSI outcome? Middle East Fertil Soc J. 2006; 11(2):99-103.
4. Mitwally MF, Abdel Razed S, Casper RF. Human chorionic gonadotrophin administration is associated with high pregnancy rates during ovarian stimulation and timed intercourse or IUI. Reprod Bio Endocrinol. 2004;2:55.
5. Gidley-Baird AA, O'Neill C, Sinosich MJ, Porter RN, Pike IL, Saunders DM. Failure of implantation in human in vitro fertilization and embryo transfer patients: the effects of altered progesterone/estrogen ratios in human and mice. Fertil Steril. 1986;45(1):69-74.
6. Forman R, Fries N, Testart J, Belaisch-Allart J, Hazout A, Frydman R. Evidence for an adverse effect of elevated serum estradiol concentrations on embryo implantation. Fertil Steril. 1988;49(1):118-22.
7. Christenson LK, Stouffer RL. Follicle stimulating hormone and luteinizing hormone/chorionic gonadotropin stimulation of vascular endothelial growth factor production by macaque granulosa cells from pre- and periovulatory follicles. J Clin Endocrinol Metab. 1997;82(7):2135-42.
8. Youssef MA, Al-Inany HG, Aboulghar M, Lam WS. Recombinant versus urinary human chorionic gonadotrophin for final oocyte maturation triggering in IVF and ICSI cycles. Cochrane Database Syst Rev. 2011;(4): CD003719.

9. Itskovitz J, Boldes R, Barlev A, Erlik Y, Kahana L, Brandes JM. The induction of LH surge and oocyte maturation by GnRH analogue (buserelin) in women undergoing ovarian stimulation for in vitro fertilization. Gynecol Endocrinol. 1988;2(Suppl 1):165.
10. Moor RM, Osborn JC, Cran OG, Walters DE. Selective effect of gonadotropins on cell coupling, nuclear maturation oocytes. Embryol Exp Morphol. 1981;61:347-65.
11. Scheele F, van der Meer M, Lambalk CB, Schoute E, Schoemaker J, Hompes PG. Exploring the recovery phase after treatment with gonadotropin-releasing hormone agonist for ovulation induction in polycystic ovary syndrome: three pilot trials. Gynecol Reprod Biol. 1995;62(2):221-4.
12. Olivennes F, Fanchin R, Bouchard P, Taieb J, Frydman R. Triggering of ovulation by gonadotropin releasing hormone agonist in patients pretreated with GnRH antagonist. Fertil Steril. 1996;66(1):151-3.
13. Cerrillo M, Rodriguez S, Mayoral M, Pacheco A, Martínez-Salazar J, Garcia-Velasco JA. Differential regulation of VEGF after final oocyte maturation with GnRH agonist versus hCG. A rationale for OHSS reduction. Fertil Steril. 2009;91(4 Suppl):1526-8.
14. Emperaire J, Ruffie A. Triggering ovulation with endogenous luteinizing hormone may prevent the ovarian hyperstimulation syndrome. Hum Reprod. 1991;6(4):506-10.
15. Monroe SE, Henzl MR, Martin MC, Schriock E, Lewis V, Nerenberg C, et al. Ablation of folliculogenesis in women by a single dose of gonadotropin-relaeasing hormone agonist: significance of time in cycle. Fertil Steril. 1985;43(3):361-8.
16. Albano C, Smitz J, Camus M. Comparison of different doses of gonadotropin-releasing hormone antagonist Cetrorelix during controlled ovarian hyperstimulation. Fertil Steril. 1997;67(5):917-22.
17. Zelinski-Wooten MB, Hutchison JS, Hess DL, Wolf DP, Stouffer RL. Follicle stimulating hormone alone supports follicle growth and oocyte development in gonadotrophin-releasing hormone antagonist-treated monkeys. Hum Reprod. 1995;10(7):1658-66
18. Meyer L, Murphy LA, Gumer A, Reichman DE, Rosenwaks Z, Cholst IN. Risk factors for a suboptimal response to gonadotropin-releasing hormone agonist trigger during in-vitro fertilization cycles. Fertil Steril. 2015;104(3): 637-42.
19. Humaidan P, Ejdrup Bredkjaer H, Westergaard LG, Andersen CY. 1,500 IU human chorionic gonadotropin administered at oocyte retrieval rescues the luteal phase when gonadotropin-releasing hormone agonist is used for ovulation induction: a prospective, randomized, controlled study. Fertil Steril. 2010;93(3):847-54.

CHAPTER 7

When to do IUI? How many Cycles of IUI?

INTRODUCTION

After the ovum is released from the follicle, it survives for maximum 6–8 hours. This may be due to tubal fluid nutrition. So, the spermatozoa must reach the ovum during this time for fertilization. Urinary luteinizing hormone (LH) kit may tell about the impending ovulation, but it cannot pinpoint the timing of intrauterine insemination (IUI). Routinely trigger is given when follicle is mature and IUI is done after 36–38 hours in majority of cases.[1] Literature shows different studies showing different timings for insemination after trigger:

- 36–38 hours
- 33–39 hours
- 18 and 42 hours
- 24 and 48 hours
- 38 hours and 24 hours later, if follicle has not ruptured.

It is documented that double IUI did not improve the pregnancy rates as compared to single IUI in the treatment of subfertile couple with husband's semen. It adds to the cost and inconvenience without adding efficacy.[2,3] Though Cantineau A et al. in Cochrane review document that double IUI may improve pregnancy rates in patients with male subfertility.[4] In all these patients, single and double IUIs were randomized and only 2D ultrasound alone was used for monitoring. Color Doppler and 3D power Doppler when used for assessing follicular maturity and endometrial receptivity, to our experience, make a significant difference in IUI results. Double IUI is to be used in a subgroup when LH surge has already started. This is explained in detail below:

Color Doppler tells about the functional maturity of the follicle. When the follicle is mature and it is the time for LH surge to start, perifollicular blood vessels show a peak systolic velocity (PSV) of 10 cm/s with RI (resistance index) <0.48. As the surge progresses, PSV shoots up and, therefore, it can be predicted that if PSV of the perifollicular vessels is high, surge has already started and follicle is closer to rupture. In an unpublished study of 350 cases of IUI, randomized for single and double IUI, it was shown that in all the patients with perifollicular PSV of more than 20 cm/s, double IUI gave significantly higher pregnancy rates, when single IUI was done at 36–38 hours after trigger and for double IUI, one IUI was done 12–14 hours after trigger and second after 36–38 hours of trigger (presented in 16th ISUOG, London, 2008) **(Fig. 1)**.

So, we recommend double IUI when PSV is ≥20 cm/s at the time of trigger. When PSV is 10 cm/s at the time of trigger, single IUI is done at 36–38 hours.

Literature support:

- Ovulation occurs between 34 and 46 hours after trigger, but the mean time interval was 38 hours.[1]
- Timing of IUI is same with human chorionic gonadotropin (hCG) or gonadotropin-releasing hormone agonists (GnRHa) trigger.[5]

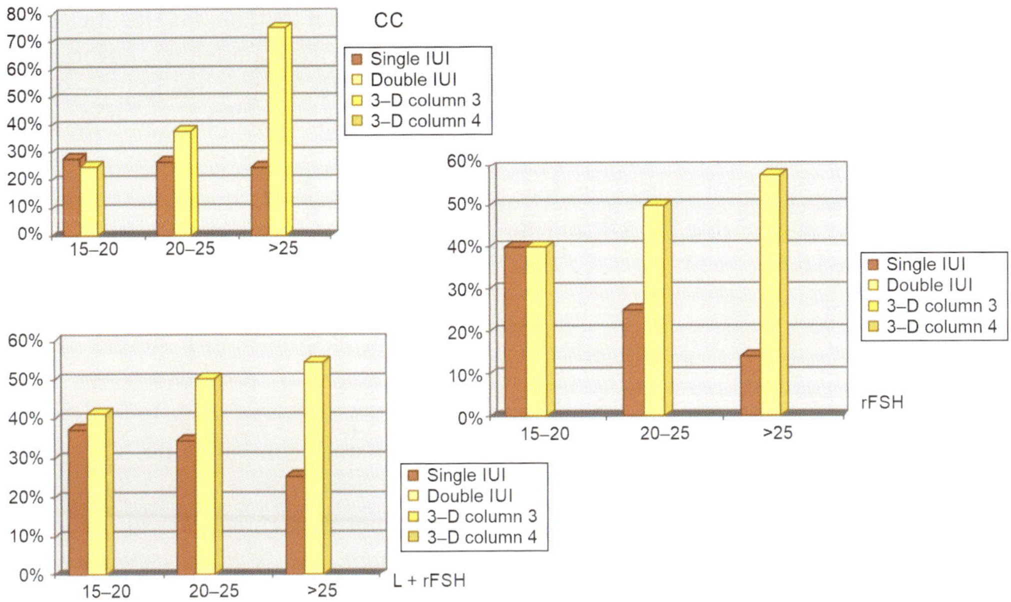

Fig. 1: Graphs showing comparative conception rates of single IUI (red columns), and double IUI (yellow columns) at different PSV values for perifollicular flow. (CC: clomiphene citrate; IUI: intrauterine insemination; rFSH: recombinant follicle-stimulating hormone)

- More pregnancies were recorded when IUI was done 12 and 34 hours after hCG than 34 and 60 hours.[6]

But, another study quotes that when all types of subfertility patients are included, double IUI has given higher pregnancy rate.[7]

Double IUI should be done in patients when pre-hCG progesterone is high, as this indicates that LH surge has started and follicle may rupture early.[8] Double IUI at 12 and 34 hours has a higher pregnancy rate.[9] Double IUI may be the answer when more follicles mature due to superovulation that are likely to rupture at different times.

Current advances in timing of IUI: Ovulation can occur within a wide timeframe ranging from 22–56 hours after the onset of LH surge. So solely based on the start of the LH surge, deciding the time of trigger is challenging. Based on several studies, optimum time for IUI in natural cycle is considered to be one day after LH surge.[10] The fertile window lasts approximately for 6 days and may vary in women with irregular cycles. So, Cochrane review concludes that timed intercourse may have higher chances of conception than IUI.[11] Chances of conception with intercourse reach 30%, 1–2 days prior to ovulation, 7% on the day of ovulation and only 1.5% on the day after ovulation.[12] A study to implement machine learning for IUI, timed intercourse or self-intracervical insemination, attributed conception to multiple factors with higher accuracy rather than relying on controversial LH surge or solely on the blood tests.[13]

Most hormonal changes including increase in LH and progesterone and decrease in estradiol take place between –1 and –2 days with some variation and it is difficult to anticipate on Day 3. Moreover, there is no definite definition of LH surge. Optimum time for IUI therefore can be considered as one day after the LH surge, most often a day before ovulation (Day 1). Conception rate is same for IUI on Day 1 or Day 2.

It was shown in ASRM practice committee report that IUI may be formal after hCG administration and upto 36 hours later with no influence on pregnancy rate, therefore IUI is done on Day 1 and Day 2. Prediction is done by E2, P and LH levels and hCG trigger is used for scheduling purposes like week ends. Based on new knowledge, artificial intelligence may replace intensive monitoring for IUI, timed intercourse or self ICI.

How many IUIs?

Intrauterine insemination is less invasive in comparison with assisted reproductive technique (ART), but IUI is always questioned for its efficacy and effectivity in comparison to ART. IUI is influenced by multiple factors. It is the least optimized procedure for infertility management. Almost all the gynecologists do IUI, but it is not standardized.

What I have observed in practice is that gynecologists do not have a good set-up of IUI and ART consultants do not believe in IUI and so is often done half-heartedly. Even if IUI is done with oral ovulogens without color Doppler monitoring, it is considered IUI failure and the technique is blamed for not giving pregnancy. But it is a person failure rather than a technique failure.

What does the literature evidence say for IUI success?

For almost all indications of IUI with mild ovarian hyperstimulation, the chances of pregnancy improve up to six cycles.[14-16] The chance of pregnancy is highest in first three cycles.[17]

There are very few studies, where more than nine cycles are attempted. Pregnancy rate after six cycles was 30% and after nine cycles, it was 41%.[18] If time is not the issue, couple should be offered nine treatment cycles especially couples in which female age is <35 years.[18]

In the same study, it was also concluded that women younger than 35 years should be offered more IUI cycles even after 6 failed attempts.

The National Institute for Healthcare and excellence fertility guidelines advocate up to six IUI cycles for patients of unexplained infertility, male subfertility, and moderate endometriosis.[19]

No evidence is found in support of offering in vitro fertilization (IVF) as a first line of treatment strategy in couples with unexplained infertility. IUI-COH (controlled ovarian hyperstimulation) should remain the treatment of first choice in these cases.[20]

So, this study contradicts the NICE guidelines and recommends immediate IVF, if patient does not conceive with expectant management. IVF is more expensive than IUI-COH without being significantly more effective. Evidence-based systematic review suggests IVF was not more effective than gonadotropins with IUI.[21] The evidence of financial, economical, and clinical consideration presented in this commentary strongly favors IUI as the first-line treatment for subfertility. Importantly, there is a need to develop global guidelines and inclusion policies for IUI and IVF procedures. These suggestions may provide sound basis for conducting the provision of publicly funded fertility services and efficient IUI practice would release Government funded fertility clinics to concentrate more on the patients who require IVF. National funding strategies should include IUI for most first-line treatment options and the UK NICE guidelines, 2013 need a radical review of IUI procedure.[22]

Only 4% of gynecologists favored NICE guideline, otherwise all believe in trying IUI before IVF after expectant management failure. IUI has a place in the era of ART as well, which the current generation of infertility specialists trained in advances in ART need to be aware of to opt for with wisdom and discretions.

The international guidelines (ESHRE, 2001; NICE, 2004; ASRM, 2012) recommend starting with less invasive treatment such as IUI and moving on to more aggressive interventions such as IVF, if these are unsuccessful or when woman is older and duration of subfertility is longer.[23]

A recent review of 2016 on assisted reproduction in male subfertility included 10 randomized controlled trials (RCTs) (757 couples). The quality of evidence was low for all comparisons. There was no difference in live birth rates between IVF/ICSI versus IUI in natural or stimulated cycles. There was no difference in terms of live births, pregnancy, or multiple pregnancy and miscarriages.[24]

Two cycles of IUI at 38–39 years give reasonable pregnancy rate and one cycle, if the age >40 years before doing IVF.[25]

Evans MB et al. in 2024 found that clinical pregnancy rate are satisfactory upto 8 consecutive OS-IUI treatment cycles. These data are useful for counseling, especially in these patients for whom in vitro fertilization is not financially or ethically feasible.[26] So many studies have documented six cycles are cost effective than IVF and in this study author has concluded that clinical pregnancy rates remain stable beyond 6 cycles. They have recorded cumulative pregnancy rate of 74% in the population. The recent study by Muthigi et al. clinical pregnancy rate are consistent with upto 6 cycles of IUI with a mean clinical pregnancy rate of 17.5%.[27] One of the explanations of higher pregnancy rate may be due to gonadotropin in 5–8 cycles, which may be refractory group.

AUTHOR'S OPINION

I fully agree that six cycles of IUI with full optimization of all steps of IUI from selection of patients to luteal support, should be tried before taking the patient for ART. But, the pregnancy rate quoted in above studies is low because in all the patients, gonadotropins were not used for ovulation induction and color Doppler was not at all used for monitoring. If these two things are added in protocol, pregnancy rate drastically increases. We can achieve pregnancy rate up to 85% in six cycles with gonadotropins and excellent ultrasound monitoring as discussed in this book. Till today when I am writing this manuscript, we have 189 patients who have conceived with IUI after three IVF failures. I have not counted one or two failures, as it is very common for the patients coming to our center. So, my carry home message is not to underestimate IUI. Do it with gonadotropins with color Doppler with excellent preparation and good luteal support. Unlike many other countries, no financial support by insurance company or government is given for infertility treatment in our country and so simpler and less expensive methods of ART should be tried sincerely to get excellent results for all patients.

CARRY HOME MESSAGE

- Single IUI is done between 36 and 38 hours.
- Double IUI is done when perifollicular PSV is >20 cm/s.
- Double IUI gives better results in male infertility.
- IUI is preferred over IVF as first line of treatment.
- At least six cycles of IUI should be done in females ≤35 years of age.
- Majority of the females conceive in 3 months with IUI.
- In younger patients, up to nine cycles of IUI should be tried.

REFERENCES

1. Andersen AG, Als-Neilsen B, Hornnes PJ, Franch Andersen L. Time interval from human

chorionic gondotrophin (hCG) injection to follicular rupture. Hum Reprod. 1995;10(12): 3202-5.
2. Polyzos NP, Tzioras S, Mauri D, Tatsioni A. Double versus single intrauterine insemination for unexplained infertility: a meta-analysis of randomized trials. Fertil Steril. 2010;94(4):1261-6.
3. Bagis T, Haydardedeoglu B, Kilcdag EB, Cok T, Simsek E, Parlakgumus AH. Single versus double intrauterine insemination in multi-follicular ovarian hyperstimulation cycles: a randomized trial. Hum Reprod. 2010;25(7): 1684-90.
4. Cantineau AEP, Heineman MJ, Cohlen BJ. Single versus double intrauterine insemination in stimulated cycles for subfertile couples. Cochrane Database Syst Rev. 2003;(1): CD003854.
5. Cantineau AEP, Janssen MJ, Cohlen BJ. Synchronized approach for intrauterine insemination in subfertile couples. Cochrane Database Syst Rev. 2014;(12):CD006942.
6. Rahman SM, Karmakar D, Malhotra N, Kumar S. Timing of intrauterine insemination: an attempt to unravel the enigma. Arch Gynecol Obstet. 2011;284(4):1023-7.
7. Astrid EP, Cantineau AEP, Cohlen BJ. Factors influencing IUI outcome: timing and number of insemination per cycle. In: Cohlen BJ, Ombelet W (Eds). Intrauterine insemination: Evidence based guidelines for daily practice. Oxford: CRC Press, Taylor and Francis Group; 2014. pp. 67-70.
8. Refnena A, Cruj M, Pacheco A. Ongoing pregnancy rates in IUI affected by late follicular phase progesterone level. Fertil Steril. 2015;104(4):879-83.
9. Ragni G, Maggioni P, Guermandi E, Testa A, Baroni E, Colombo M, et al. Efficacy of double intrauterine insemination in controlled ovarian hyperstimulation cycles. Fertil Steril. 1999;72(4):619-22.
10. Cohlen B, Bijkerk A, Van Der Poel S, Van der Veen F, van Wely M. Intrauterine insemination review and systematic assessment of the evidence that supports global recommendations. Hum Reprod Update. 2018;24:300-19.
11. Manders M, Mclindon L, Schluze B, Beckmann MM, Kremer JA, Farquhar C. Timed intercourse for couples trying to conceive. Cochrane Database Syst Rev. 2015:CD011345.
12. Stanford JB, White JL, Hatasaka H. Timing intercourse to achieve pregnancy: current evidence. Obstet Gynecol. 2002;100:1333-41.
13. Youngster M, Luz A, Baum M, Hourvitz R, Reuvenny S, Maman E, Hourvitz A. Artificial intelligence in the service of intrauterine insemination and timed intercourse in spontaneous cycles. Fertil Steril. 2023;120(5): 1004-11.
14. Bensdrop A, Cohlen BJ, Heineman MJ, Vanderkerchove P. Intrauterine insemination for male subfertility. Cochrane Database Sys Rev. 2007;(3):CD000360.
15. Goverde AJ, McDonnel J, Vermeiden JPW, Schats R, Rutten FF, Schoemaker J. Intrauterine insemination or in-vitro fertilization in idiopathic subfertility: a randomized trial and cost-effectiveness analysis. Lancet. 2000; 355(9197):13-8.
16. Merviel P, Heraud MH, Grenier N, Lourdel E, Sanguinet P, Copin H. Predictive factors for pregnancy after intrauterine insemination(IUI): an analysis of 1038 cycles and a review of literature. Fertil Steril. 2010:93(1):79-88.
17. Aboulghar M, Mansour R, Serour G, Abdrazek A, Amin Y, Rhodes C. Controlled ovarian hyper-stimulation and intrauterine insemination for treatment of unexplained infertility should be limited to maximum of three trials. Fertil Steril. 2001:75(1):88-91.
18. Custers IM, Steures P, Hompes P, Flierman P, van Kasteren Y, van Dop PA, et al. Intrauterine insemination: how many cycles should we perform? Hum Reprod. 2008;23(4):885-8.
19. National Institute for Health and Care Excellence. Fertility Assessment and Treatment of People with Infertility Problems. Clinical Guidelines CG 11. London: NICE; 2004. [online] Available from https://www.nice.org.uk/guidance/CG11. [Last accessed November, 2020].
20. Tjon-Kon-Fat RI, Bensdorp AJ, Bossuyt PMM, Koks C, Oosterhuis GJE, Hoek A, et al. Is IVF-served two different ways—more cost effective than IUI with controlled ovarian hyper-stimulation? Hum Reprod. 2015;30(10):2331-9.
21. Gunn DD, Bates GW. Evidence-based approach to unexplained infertility: a systematic review. Fertil Steril. 2016;105(6):1566-74.
22. Bahadur G, Homburg R, Muneer A, Tacuch P, Alangaden T, Al-Habib A, et al. First line fertility treatment strategies regarding IUI and IVF require clinical evidence. Hum Reprod. 2016;31(6):1141-6.
23. Van den Boogaard NM. Prognostic profiles and effectiveness of assisted conception: secondary analysis of individual patient's data. Hum Reprod Update. 2014;20(1):141-51.

24. Cissen M, Bensdrop A, Cohlen BJ, Repping S, de Bruin JP, van Wely M. Assisted reproductive technologies for male subfertility. Cochrane Database Syst Rev. 2016;(2):CD000360.
25. Harris ID, Missmer SA, Hornstein MD. Poor success of gonadotropin induced controlled ovarian hyperstimulation and intrauterine insemination for older women. Fertil Steril. 2010;94:144-8.
26. Evans MB, Hosseinzadeh P, Flannagan K, Jahandideh S, Buruss E, Peck JD, et al. Assesment of clinical pregnancies in upto eight ovarian stimulation with intrauterine insemination treatment cycles in those unable to proceed with in vitro fertilization. Fertil Steril. 2024;122(1):114-20.
27. Muthigi A, Jahandideh S, Bishop LA, Naemmi FK, Shipley SK, O'Brein JE, et al. Clarifying the relationship between total mobile sperm counts and intrauterine insemination pregnancy rates. Fertil Steril. 2021;115:1454-60.

CHAPTER 8

Technique of Intrauterine Insemination

INTRODUCTION

I am doing intrauterine insemination (IUI) since about 30 years. In 1992, I learnt IUI from the experts of Bourne Hall clinic. As the time passed with experience and self-audit, we adapted several modifications in the semen wash technique, in IUI procedure, in the drugs used, over and above what we had learnt as principles of IUI. In this chapter, I am going to discuss exactly what I am doing for my IUI patients. It may not match to what has been documented in other literature, but still I will be honest with you all and describe here exactly what I am doing. And, I am very confident about my technique and methodology because I have more than 10,500 pregnancies with IUI in patients with long-term infertility.

PREPROCEDURE PREPARATION

Intrauterine insemination laboratory should be as close to the IUI room as possible (possibly adjacent). The prepared sample should be inseminated as soon as it is ready. Patient is placed in lithotomy position. Full bladder or half full bladder is absolutely not necessary. It may be advised in acutely anteverted uterus. We do not clean the vagina with saline or Ringer's lactate or any antiseptic agent. Though vagina is to be evaluated early in the cycle at any time to exclude vaginal infection, especially if the history suggests so. If there was infection in the vagina, it is to be treated by proper medicines to cure it before IUI.

TECHNIQUE OF INTRAUTERINE INSEMINATION

Place Sims speculum and hold the anterior lip of cervix with Alyce's forceps after retracting the anterior vaginal wall with retractor. Hold Alyce's forceps in such a way that you can support your little finger just above symphysis pubis, in a similar way that is done while dilating the cervix. This helps to bring the endometrial cavity and the cervical canal in a straight line. The argument here may be that using Alyce's forceps may stimulate uterine contractions, but to my opinion that is not a problem, because it may lead to closing of the cornual ends and thus reduce the amount on intratubal insemination is only theoretical. A low frequency and high intensity of uterine contractions on the day of IUI appear to be associated with higher pregnancy rates.[1] In one of the trials, using tenaculum to hold the cervix has increased the pregnancy rates, whereas uterine relaxants before IUI have not improved pregnancy rates.[1]

Then introduce IUI cannula and allow it to pass across the internal os. You may release the prepared semen sample in the endometrial cavity. It is not essential to go beyond the mid-cavity of the uterus. One should not advance the cannula to may touch the fundus of the endometrial cavity and then withdraw the cannula back and then inject. This can damage the endometrium and bleeding may occur. Cannulas with side holes are available and they are marketed by the argument that the side holes allow the flow of the prepared semen sample directly into the tube. This is not a valid argument and direct flow of the fluid in the tube is not required. In fact, it may wash the ovum out of the tube.

Uterus can hold only 0.4 mL of fluid in its cavity. If it is injected in excess, it flows into the fallopian tubes or may flow out through the cervix into vagina. We usually inject 0.5-0.7 mL of the prepared (washed) semen sample and so there is almost always some intratubal insemination. This is the reason that when the washed semen sample is being inseminated, one should be very slow and gentle. Since there is some amount of intratubal insemination almost always with intrauterine insemination, the results are similar to that of "GIFT" (gamete intra-fallopian tube transfer). Therefore "GIFT" is no more practiced.

As excess amount of the prepared sample, beyond 0.4–0.5 mL, flows out of the vagina, patient always complains of fluid dribbling out through the vagina and blames that for negative results. It is therefore essential to counsel the patient for this purpose.

After the procedure, 15 minutes of rest is sufficient in the lying down position. Head low position or elevation of the buttocks with pillow is not required. After 15 minutes, the patient can do all her routine activities, no further rest is required. Normal transportation time from intracervical insemination to fallopian tube is 2–10 minutes and so whatever the position of the woman, sperms usually reach the tube immediately after IUI. But cumulative pregnancy rate is higher, if immobilization for 10–15 minutes is done after IUI rather than immediate mobilization. But resting beyond that time does not increase pregnancy rates.[2,3]

TIPS AND CONTRADICTIONS

The instruments in the tray include Sims' speculum, single catch Alyce's forceps, and anterior vaginal wall retractor. We do not use Cusco's speculum because in my experience when using Cusco's speculum, there is a difficulty in passage of the cannula across the internal os in about 20–30% of cases. This is because majority of the patients presenting with infertility are nulliparous and the cervix is high, at times above the ischial spine with acute curve between cervix and uterus. In several of these cases, advancing the cannula without damaging the internal os is not possible. Apart from damage, the manipulation required also leads to more time from semen preparation to injection. And, it is documented in literature that the success of IUI is affected by the amount of manipulation that has to be done during IUI.

Endometrial scratching during follicular phase of same cycle of IUI with flexible aspiration catheter may improve ongoing pregnancy rate and standardization of technique is required. But majority of the studies in IVF are not found to be useful.[4]

There is always a confusion on the part of the couple whether to keep relations before IUI or not. They should be allowed intercourse at any time during the follicular phase. Long abstinence will have dead sperms and pus cells in the semen sample. Abstinence of <2 days usually gives higher pregnancy rate. We always ask the patient to have an intercourse on the day of trigger and then the sample for IUI is collected on the day of IUI.[5]

SITE OF INSEMINATION IN DONOR INSEMINATION

Pregnancy rate per cycle in cryopreserved sperms is always less than fresh sperms.[6] (The recent Cochrane review suggests high pregnancy rate for IUI with ovarian hyperstimulation compared to intracervical insemination with ovarian hyperstimulation.[7] Ovarian stimulation can cause multiple pregnancy rate and as the woman is not subfertile in donor insemination cycles, ovarian hyperstimulation may be avoided to avoid multiple pregnancies.

Difficulty in introduction of catheter:

- Hold the cervix with a single tooth Alyce's forceps and in majority of patients, the passage of IUI cannula is easy.
- Cervical mucus is always good, provided the follicle quality is good. So, use Doppler to assess the follicular quality.
- Curved cannula can help in acutely anteverted or retroflexed uterus.
- If all efforts fail, tip of tuberculin syringe is introduced through external os. It should be pushed so that maximum possible distance in cervix it penetrates and then slowly 0.8–1 mL of prepared semen sample is injected. 0.3–0.5 mL will definitely reach the endometrial cavity if internal os is open. Rest of the amount may spill off. Fairly good pregnancy rate can be achieved by this maneuver, rather than wasting the cycle.
- Prophylactic antibiotic does not have a role.

Occasionally, when patient is not co-operative after all the efforts, IUI under anesthesia may be required. I had to do this in about five patients in my practice period of 25 years, which means it is rarely required.

When uterine contractions are seen frequently, pregnancy rate and live birth rate increases. Myometrial contractions are necessary for achieving fertilization, as these allow the sperms to go to fallopian tube.[8]

Singleton live birth rate with one cycle of IVF was not significantly different than three cycles of IUI with controlled ovarian hyper-stimulation with gonadotropins.[9] So, IVF is not regarded as first line of treatment.[10]

CARRY HOME MESSAGE

- Intrauterine insemination should be done as early as possible after semen preparation.
- Using Sims' speculum and Alyce's forceps for IUI does not affect the results negatively.
- 10–15 minutes of immobilization after IUI gives better pregnancy rate.
- Abstinence is not advised before IUI.

REFERENCES

1. Swierkowski N, Boitrelle F, Alter L, Selva J, Quibel T, Torre A. Uterine contractility and elastography as prognostic factors for pregnancy after intrauterine insemination. Fertil Steril. 2017;107(4):961-8.
2. Custers IM, Flierman PA, Maas P, Cox T, Van Dessel TJHM, Gerards MH, et al. Immobilization versus immediate mobilization after intrauterine insemination: Randomized controlled trial. BMJ. 2009;339:b4080.
3. Saleh A, Tan SL, Biljan MM, Tulandi T. A randomized study of the effect of 10 minutes of bedrest after intrauterine insemination. Fertil Steril. 2000;74(3):509-11.
4. Vitegliana A, Noventa M, Saccone G, Gizzo S, Vitale SG, Laganà AS, et al. Endometrial scratch injury before IUI: is it time to re-evalaute its value? Evidence from a systematic review and meta-analysis of randomized controlled trials. Fertil Steril. 2018;109(1):84-96.
5. Marshburu PB, Alanis M, Matthews ML, Usadi R, Papadakis MH, Kullstam S, et al. Short period of ejaculatory abstinence before intra-uterine insemination is associated with higher pregnancy rate. Fertil Steril. 2010;93(1):286-9.
6. Subak LL, Adamson D, Boltz NL. Therapeutic Donor insemination. A prospective rando-mized trial of fresh versus frozen sperm. Am J Obstet Gyencol. 1992;166(6 Pt 1):1597-604.
7. Besselink DE, Farquhar C, Kremer JAM, Majoribanks J, O'Brien P. Cervical insemination versus intrauterine insemination of donor sperm for subfertility. Cochrane Database Syst Rev. 2009;(2):CD000317.
8. Blasco V, Prados N, Carranza F, González-Ravina C, Pellicer A, Fernández-Sánchez M. Influence of follicle rupture and uterine contractions on IUI outcome: a new predictive model. Fertil Steril. 2014;102(4):1034-40.
9. Nandi A, Bhide P, Hooper R, Shah A, Khan K, Homburg R, et al. IUI with gonadotrophin stimulation or IVF for treatment of unexplained subfertility. Fertil Steril. 2017;107(2):1329-35.
10. Tjon-Kon-Fit RI, Bensdorp AJ, Bossuyt PMM, Koks C, Oosterhuis GJE, Hoek A, et al. Is IVF-Served two different ways-more cost effective than IUI with controlled ovarian hyperstimulation? Hum Reprod. 2015;30(10): 2331-9.

CHAPTER 9

Luteal Phase Support for Intrauterine Insemination

INTRODUCTION

Luteal phase support is an equally important step for the success of intrauterine insemination (IUI). Luteal support is required in IUI cycles from the day of IUI or from the following day, and it improves the pregnancy rate.[1]

When to use the luteal phase support in IUI?

- Natural cycle
- Clomiphene citrate (CC)
- Letrozole
- Gonadotropin stimulation
- Gonadotropin-releasing hormone (GnRH) agonist protocol
- GnRH antagonist protocol
- GnRH agonist trigger

Natural Cycle

There are some centers in the world where luteinizing hormone (LH) surge is detected by LH urinary kit and IUI is done. No gonadotropins or human chorionic gonadotropin (hCG) or antagonists are given in the cycle. In natural cycle, when follicle develops, E2 is >150 pgm/mL/follicle. This E2 is sufficient to develop progesterone receptors and to cause positive feedback for LH release. This high LH lasts for >48 hours and is enough to rescue the corpus luteal function. These follicle-stimulating hormone (FSH) and LH surge last for about 48 hours. The LH surge has a short ascending phase of 14 hours, a peak plateau of 20 hours and descending phase of 20 hours. This LH surge is sufficient to maintain luteal phase and so routine use of progesterone in luteal phase is not justified in natural unstimulated cycles.[2] So, routine use of progesterone is not justified in natural cycle. Progesterone is therefore not routinely started after spontaneous rupture of the follicle.

The cause of luteal phase defect (LPD) in natural nonassisted reproduction technology (ART) cycles is abnormal folliculogenesis. Unhealthy follicle that produces less E2, leading to less progesterone receptors and lower peak of LH. This lower LH peak will give unhealthy corpus luteum and low progesterone levels. The clinical situations when LH surge is inadequate are:

- Hypoprolactinemia
- Extremes of age
- Stress
- Polycystic ovary syndrome (PCOS)
- Endometriosis
- Obesity
- Anorexia
- Athletes
- Postpartum
- Infections

Hypothalamic-pituitary dysfunction disturbs GnRH pulsatility, which in-turn disturbs FSH and LH secretion, which leads to abnormal folliculogenesis and LPD. So, all these patients require ovulation induction to improve the quality of the follicle. But pregnancy is only 2–8% in IUI in natural cycle and so natural cycle IUI is not routinely practical in India.

Luteal Phase Support with Clomiphene Citrate

Clomiphene acts on hypothalamus and pituitary to secrete FSH and LH that leads to development of follicles and secretes more estrogen. High estrogen causes upregulation of LH and progesterone receptors. Therefore, in clomiphene-stimulated cycles, LPD is not common. In spite of estrogen receptors being occupied by CC, multiple follicles develop and there is no abnormality of LH or progesterone secretion because of high E2 level. LPD found in CC cycle is due to high LH, particularly in polycystic ovarian syndrome (PCOS) patients, that is detrimental to ovum leading to abnormal folliculogenesis and is responsible for LPD. Adding estrogen to clomiphene is not proved to improve the pregnancy rate. So, luteal phase support is not justified in clomiphene cycles.[3,4]

Luteal Support in Letrozole Cycle

Letrozole prevents aromatization of androgen to estrogen leading to estrogen deficiency. This E2 deficiency has negative feedback to pituitary causing release of FSH and LH, which develops follicle. E2 from developed follicle goes to pituitary and decreases FSH and LH to give monofollicular development. This decrease in LH may cause LPD and decrease in E2 may lead to poor development of progesterone receptors. Therefore, when letrozole is used for ovulation induction, luteal phase support is indicated, though sufficient literature on the same is still not available. Luteal support with vaginal progesterone increases clinical pregnancy rate in women with PCOS using letrozole for ovulation induction.[5]

Luteal Phase Support in Gonadotropin Cycle

Exogenous gonadotropins affect the ovaries to produce more E2. This leads to negative feedback to hypothalamic-pituitary ovarian (HPO) axis and may lead to abnormal LH pulsatility and abnormal progesterone secretion from corpus luteum.[6] Though progesterone is important for pregnancy, elevated progesterone level on the day of trigger affects pregnancy rates adversely. Progesterone level of 1.5 ng/mL is a threshold for poor ovarian responders, >1.75 ng/mL is associated with low ongoing pregnancy rates for intermediate responders, and 2.25 ng/mL can be applied for high responders.[7] This progesterone level is elevated in superovulated cycles, as each mature follicle secretes a trace of progesterone. Endometrium is exposed to progesterone before hCG injection leads to decreased endometrial receptivity.[8] A systematic review and meta-analysis suggest that luteal phase support improved the likelihood of clinical pregnancy and live birth in gonadotropin-stimulated IUI cycles.[1]

It is an established fact that luteal phase is defective in all stimulated cycles.[9] In controlled ovarian stimulation, there are multiple follicles, which grow giving supraphysiological levels of E2 and progesterone, which inhibits LH secretion by the pituitary by negative feedback at hypothalamic-pituitary axis level for LH release, which causes early demise of corpus luteum and fall in progesterone level.[10] Moreover, agonist or antagonist has already suppressed LH in follicular phase and therefore endogenous LH is very low. Adequate LH is important for maintenance of corpus luteum. So, luteal phase support is required in all the patients when agonists or antagonists are used. Endogenous LH is also important for secretion of other growth factors and cytokines and leukemia inhibitory factor (LIF) for implantation. Exogenous hCG helps to rescue corpus luteum. In gonadotropin stimulation, there is advancement of histology in late proliferative phase, earlier shift into implantation window, and asynchrony if the maturation of mid and late luteal phase due to high E2, i.e., altered E2/P ratio.[11]

So, in all gonadotropin stimulated cycles, luteal phase support is mandatory. We do all our cycles of IUI with gonadotropins or letrozole with gonadotropins and so we give luteal support to all these patients.

Luteal Support with hCG Trigger

In follicular phase, LH is low because of agonist or antagonist as well as high E2 and progesterone giving negative feedback to pituitary for LH. However, early luteal phase function of LH is covered by bolus of hCG (5,000–10,000 IU), which is routinely used for trigger. hCG also secures growth factor and cytokines for implantation. Normally, 500 IU of hCG is required for completion of meiosis and 9,500 IU of hCG is required for follicular rupture. Therefore, in intrauterine insemination (IUI) cycles, usually 10,000 IU of hCG is given. But, this dose may be too large for assisted reproductive technology (ART) cycles. But, this large dose takes care of the corpus luteum in the early luteal phase and maintains progesterone secretion from corpus luteum. The hCG supports corpus luteum only for 5 days and the embryo starts producing hCG after 8th day after ovulation that will again support the corpus luteum. So, from 5th to till 8th day, corpus luteum is not supported and there is progesterone deficiency, and it is known as "luteal gap" and leads to implantation failure or early abortions.[12]

After Day 5, endogenous LH levels are also low due to high surrogate LH and high progesterone.[13] It is crucial to have certain amplitude and frequency of LH during the luteal phase. Progesterone supplement is therefore essential for the luteal phase support when hCG trigger is given.[14]

To decide the time of IUI, we always give trigger, and it is mostly hCG. Luteal support is essential in all the patients when hCG is given as trigger.

Luteal Phase Support in Agonist Cycle

Gonadotropin-releasing hormone agonists are not used for downregulation in IUI cycles. These increase the cost as the requirement of gonadotropins is increased and can also lead to multiple pregnancies and ovarian hyperstimulation syndrome (OHSS).[15]

Luteal Support in Antagonist Cycle

It is especially used in thin lean PCOS patients and luteal support is a must.

The antagonist is started from the day the lead follicle reaches 14 mm. It suppresses the LH level temporarily before ovulation trigger. It was formerly believed that antagonist cycles do not require luteal phase support and so lots of pregnancies were wasted. But then, it was understood that suppression of LH by antagonist also continues in the luteal phase, and it reduces luteal phase length and compromises pregnancy rate. Antagonist downregulation decreases the risk of OHSS and does allow the use of agonist as a trigger, thus almost abolishing the risk of OHSS.

GnRHa Trigger

In PCOS, we use chronic low-dose protocol and calculate the dose of gonadotropin from the dose chart[16] and, therefore, there is less chance of multiple follicle recruitment. In spite of that if multiple follicles develop, there is a risk of OHSS, if hCG is given as a trigger. In these patients, GnRH agonist is used for trigger. GnRHa causes FSH and LH surge, while hCG causes only LH surge. FSH surge is a must in animals for completion of meiosis of the ovum and rupture of the follicle, but its role in human being is not yet fully understood. LH surge that occurs after GnRHa trigger completes meiosis but may be inadequate for the luteal support and thus leads to LPD. LH surge that occurs after GnRHa has only 4 hours of ascending limb and 14 hours of descending limb, whereas the natural LH surge has an ascending limb of 14 hours, plateau of 20 hours, and descending limb of 20 hours. This difference in time of action between the two cannot be bridged by increasing the dose of GnRHa, as the defect is because of low LH. At least 600 mg/day of exogenous progesterone is required to support luteal phase in these patients.

STRATEGIES FOR SUPPORTING LUTEAL PHASE AFTER GnRHa TRIGGER

- Exogenous E2 + P support with close monitoring
- *Dual trigger:* Agonist + hCG (1,000–2,500 IU)
- hCG 1,500 IU at the time of IUI
- Low-dose hCG in luteal phase
- Luteal phase LH administration

- *Intensive luteal support*: Intramuscular (IM) progesterone 25–75 mg/day or micronized progesterone 800 mg/day vaginally with estradiol patch 0.1 mg, 3–4, on alternate days or 2–8 mg with oral estradiol valerate is given. Adjust the dose to keep serum E2 level >200 pgm/mL and progesterone level 20 ng/mL by frequent testing. The results are similar to those of hCG trigger and progesterone support.[17]
- *Dual trigger: Agonist + hCG (1,000–2,500 IU):* Along with GnRHa trigger, hCG 1,000–2,500 IU is added for rescuing CL by providing additional signal for adequate luteinization. It has given pregnancy rate up to 53% with one case of OHSS.[18] If serum E2 is <1,600 pgm/mL, GnRHa trigger with 1,000–2,500 IU of hCG gives good pregnancy rates with almost no risk of OHSS. The other advantage of dual trigger is that sometimes LH peak may not be sufficient with agonist trigger and if it is <9 IU/mL, meiosis may not occur. Adding low-dose hCG with agonist assures meiosis.
- *hCG at the time of IUI:* When pretrigger E2 is <1,600 pgm/mL or when there are <25 follicles of >11 mm in diameter, hCG 1,500 IU is given at the time of IUI to rescue the corpus luteum and achieve comparable pregnancy rates to hCG trigger. Second bolus is not given, as it may increase the risk of OHSS.[9] So, modified luteal phase support may be GnRHa trigger, hCG 1,500 IU after IUI, vaginal micronized progesterone 400 mg BD and E2 2 mg, and BD supplementation. This regimen reduces OHSS and gives more eggs with equal live birth rates.[9]
- *Low-dose beta-hCG:* 100–150 IU hCG as luteal support is enough to rescue the corpus luteum and produce sufficient progesterone for adequate luteal support.[19] In the same paper, it has also been mentioned that it causes blood levels of progesterone as high as 10–15 IU/L, which is sufficient for mid-luteal phase and is similar to 6,500 IU of hCG for ovulation trigger and vaginal progesterone. But delivery of this small dose of hCG is difficult at present. This might prove to be a choice of luteal phase support, if hCG becomes available in Pen device.
- *Recombinant LH:* It is very useful, as it lowers the incidence of OHSS. But it is very expensive and, therefore, its usage is not accepted in clinical practice.

Whenever agonist trigger is given, estradiol valerate 2 mg BD should be given to all patients, as corpus luteum does not secrete E2 in sufficient amount. The standard dose of estradiol valerate is 2 mg BD.

What to give for luteal support?

For luteal support in IUI, we can give progesterone and/or hCG. Let us evaluate both the drugs:

Progesterone

Natural micronized progesterone is the most common drug used for luteal phase support in IUI. It can be given by:

1. Vaginal route:
   - *Vaginal suppositories*: Vaginal application is the most accepted route for progesterone administration. It has several advantages:

     Natural micronized progesterone:
     - Reduced size
     - Enhances dissolution
     - Maximum serum concentration
     - Reduced destruction
     - Increases half-life

   - It avoids all gastrointestinal (GI) side effects and sedative and hypnotic effects.
   - The first uterine pass effect (FUPE) **(Fig. 1)** is another major advantage: From the vagina, the drug is directly transported to the uterus. So, in spite of low blood levels of progesterone, its level in uterus is high. Migration of the drug occurs from cervix and lower segment of uterus to the fundus of the uterus.[15] A countercurrent exchange **(Fig. 2)** also occurs in the upper third of the vagina. The drug is absorbed in the veins of the vagina and from there directly goes to the arteries of the uterus, without entering into the general circulation. This leads to low-serum level but high concentration in the uterus.[16-18]

   These mechanisms lead to consistent tissue level of progesterone with vaginal application.[15] In spite of low-blood levels, this improves implantation rates and decreases early pregnancy loss.[9]

   Czajkowski et al. proved that vaginal progesterone 300 mg is effective in reducing spiral artery pulsatility, PI, and S/D ratio as compared to 30 mg of oral dydrogesterone.[19] Ahmed Mohammed et al. have found in their study of systematic review and meta-analysis of RCT vaginal versus IM progesterone for luteal support in ART that vaginal progesterone has same results as IM progesterone in ART and is more satisfactory.[20,21]

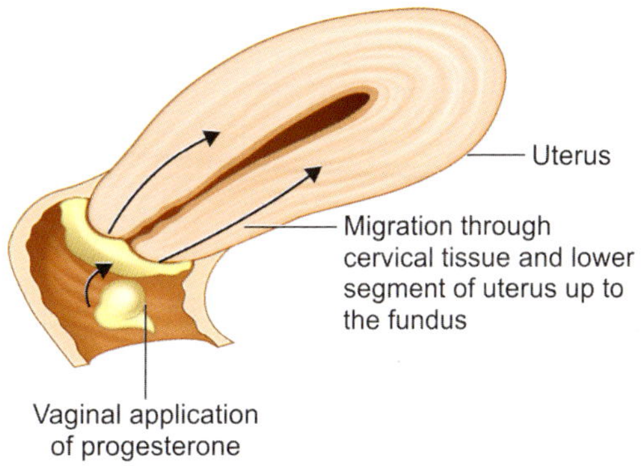

Fig. 1: Diagrammatic representation of uterine first-pass effect.

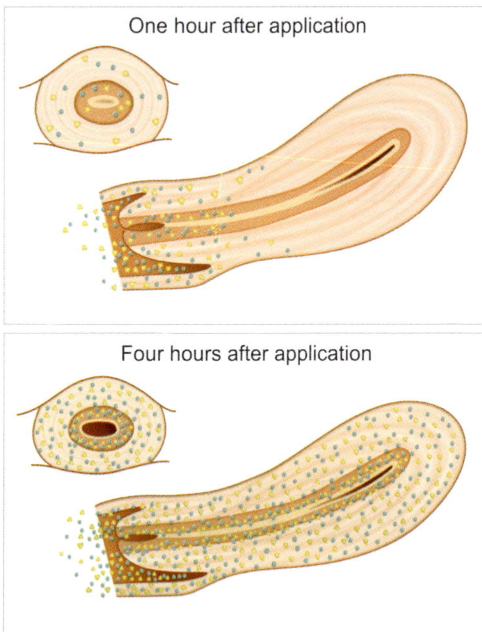

Fig. 2: Progressive diffusion of progesterone from the cervix to the fundus of the uterus.

- *Progesterone vaginal effervescent tablets:* This is a new delivery system of progesterone. Disintegration of tablet occurs in 7–10 minutes. It increases absorption. Twice a day dosage can achieve higher concentration of progesterone and reach steady state within 24–32 hours and maintain mean concentration above 10 ng/mL.[22]

  As explained in **Figure 3**, the absorption of progesterone occurs by passive diffusion as well as paracellular transport, which results in greater concentration and prolonged blood levels. CO_2 opens up tight junctions of the cells and so paracervical absorption is increased.

  Advantages of effervescent tablet:
  - Greater bioavailability
  - Effective systemic absorption
  - Avoids hepatic first-pass metabolism
  - Higher concentration in endometrium
  - Lower doses are required.
  - Less fluctuation in serum levels
  - Healthy vaginal environment because of acidic pH
    - As efficient as other vaginal progesterone
    - Less irritation and discharge
- *Vaginal progesterone rings:* These are also available now. These rings once inserted would release 10–20 nmol/L for 90 days. Compared to 50 mg/day IM progesterone, this product has shown comparable or better implantation rate.[22]

2. *Oral tablets:*
   - It is available as soft gelatin capsules or tablet form and as sustained release tablets.
   - It causes drowsiness, flushing, and nausea and it has selective and hypnotic effects because of metabolites.
   - It causes fluid retention.
   - Efficacy changes with food particle size and its vehicle. Bioavailability is only 10% when taken orally.
   - Extensive first-pass hepatic metabolism and therefore multiple doses are required. It has poor intestinal absorption.
   - It is ineffective in inducing an in-phase secretory endometrium.[12]
   - It has a lower pregnancy rate.

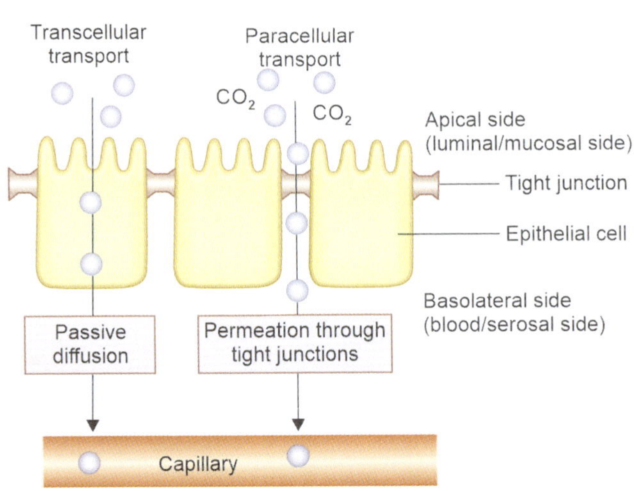

Fig. 3: Diagrammatic explanation of the vaginal absorption of effervescent progesterone vaginal tablets (from monogram Susten VT).

Oral sustained release tablets: Slow release (SR) EROMAT is a new technology. The drug is released gradually in a controlled manner over a span of 16–24 hours in the distal part of the GI tract allowing lymphatic absorption of intact drug into systematic circulation and direct entry of the drug through the mucosal lining of colon into systemic circulation. The dose of sustained release progesterone capsule is 200–400 mg daily. This has less side effects compared to conventional oral preparation. Only 20% of the drug is released in the first 4 hours and minimizes hepatic and prehepatic metabolism. Rest of the drug is released in distal GI tract. The serum *P* level should be >14 ng/mL for threatened abortion and LPD. Oral SR preparations, 400/300/200 mg/day, give blood levels up to 46.2/36.2/20.6 ng/mL, respectively.

The drug at present is available in very few countries and there are not many international trials available to prove its role. The sole application of this drug is not recommended by majority of the ART clinics. It is always used in combination of other progesterones. This drug still requires further studies in spite of its wide availability.

3. *Subcutaneous aqueous injections*: Subcutaneous injections have replaced intramuscular injections now. *Subcutaneous aqueous progesterone* preparations are also available now in which progesterone is combined with cyclodextrin, a starch residue, and is given as 25 mg or 50 mg doses a day and has shown results compatible with intramuscular progesterone.[13] Gillian et al. have proved that subcutaneous injection of water-soluble progesterone 25 mg is safe and as effective as vaginal progesterone gel and remains an option for those who do not want vaginal progesterone on cultural, personal, or medical reasons.[14]

   Transdermal progesterone is not the option because the skin is rich in five reductases, which will inactivate progesterone. Another reason is that daily E2 production is 0.5 mg/24 hours, while that of progesterone is 25 mg/24 hours. Such large doses are difficult to deliver by transdermal patches.
4. *Progesterone gel*: It increases the pregnancy rate in IUI.[20,21] It contains 90 mg (8%) of progesterone. It contains micronized progesterone in emulsion system, which also contains water insoluble polymer, "polycarbophil" having mucin-like actions. It is as effective as vaginal tablets. There is no substantial difference in ongoing pregnancy rate between vaginal progesterone gel and vaginal micronized progesterone tablets.[23] But vaginal gel has given higher pregnancy rates than intramuscular progesterone below the age of 35 years in IVF (in vitro fertilization) patients and after the age of 35 years, pregnancy rates were same for both the gel and the intramuscular progesterone group.[24] Its dosage schedule is once a day, so acceptance is very good. Only disadvantage of this preparation is its high cost. Gel preparation is always used in the morning and the patient is advised not to rest after that. Because of the movements, friction occurs between the vaginal walls that help to separate progesterone and facilitate its absorption. Absorption will be poor, if it is applied at night. If it is to be applied twice a day, the evening application should be at least 3–4 hours before bedtime.

Human Chorionic Gonadotropin Supplementation

In a normo-ovulatory female, in unstimulated cycle, administration of hCG in luteal phase does not downregulate LH secretion in luteal phase.[22] It stimulates theca-lutein cells to produce more progesterone and other steroids that are required for the maintenance of normal pregnancy. hCG also increases the placental protein 4 and relaxing that are required for implantation. It is administered every 3–4 days. It is given in the dosage of 2,000 IU on Day 3, 7, and 10 or 5,000 IU on Day 5–9 postovulatory. It is an excellent drug in non-in vitro fertilization (IVF) patients and in poor responders in IVF also. But, if the pretrigger E2 is >1,600 IUI cycle, hCG is not given as a trigger for the risk of OHSS. In these cases, agonist is given as a trigger and hCG 1,500 IU is given at the time of IUI to rescue the corpus luteum, if the number of follicles is not >25 of >11 mm in diameter. It gives equal pregnancy rates as hCG trigger and avoids OHSS.[23,9]

Disadvantages of hCG:

- It should not be given when E2 is >1,600 pg/mL in IUI cycles because of risk of OHSS and multiple pregnancies.
- When there are more follicles, it will increase E2 and may change E2:P, which may decrease implantation but this is only theoretical assumption.
- Even the low dose of hCG, as 1,500 IU is given, every 3 days after agonist trigger, can cause OHSS.[9]
- Prolonged hCG exposure in proliferative phase may affect endometrial receptivity.[24]
- During natural menstrual cycle, LH in luteal phase seldom exceeds 5–10 IU/mL, which is capable of eliciting progesterone level in excess of 25–35 nmol/L. So, supraphysiological levels of LH/hCG are not required in luteal phase. Endogenous progesterone is very high due to multiple corpus lutea and exogenous progesterone results in concentration of <75 nmol/L only.
  Microdose supplement 100–150 IU/day of hCG throughout the luteal phase without using any exogenous progesterone is sufficient. The progesterone level thus achieved is similar to that achieved when ovulation trigger is given by 6,500 IU hCG with progesterone support. When this microdose hCG is used with agonist trigger, hCG levels remain within physiological limits, i.e., 5–10 IU/mL. The only difficulty is the delivery of microdose.[25]

ONSET OF LUTEAL SUPPORT

It is started from the day or the day following IUI.

DURATION OF LUTEAL SUPPORT

Prospective randomized controlled trial[26] indicated that prolongation of progesterone supplementation in early pregnancy had no influence on miscarriage rate. Theoretically, we can stop progesterone support once beta-hCG is positive, but most of the infertility specialists continue till 10–12 weeks of pregnancy. Caspo et al. have shown that continuation of pregnancy is independent of corpus luteum function as early as 8–10 weeks of pregnancy.[27] The function is taken over by placenta.[28] The study by Graciela Kohls et al. has shown that vaginal progesterone supplementation after ART can be safely withdrawn at 5 weeks of gestation because cycle outcome was similar to conventional luteal support that is given till 8 weeks of gestation.[29] At 5 weeks, hCG level is >1,000 IU/L and that is sufficient to support corpus luteum. The circulating level of progesterone is >8 ng/mL at 5 weeks of pregnancy.

CARRY HOME MESSAGE

- Luteal phase defect is because of low progesterone or suboptimal response with normal progesterone.
- Low progesterone may be due to abnormal folliculogenesis in non-IVF patients.
- No laboratory tests are reliable for diagnosis of LPD.
- Corpus luteum rescue is because of hCG.
- Low progesterone is because of low hCG in unhealthy embryo.
- Duration of exposure of progesterone is important than blood levels.
- Ovulation induction is a very useful luteal support.
- Human chorionic gonadotropin is also an effective luteal support. 100–150 IU of hCG may prove to be good alternative to luteal support.
- Micronized progesterone is the best.
- Vaginal route is the best route.
- Subcutaneous route has replaced IM route.
- Luteal support in natural cycle is not justified.
- Progesterone support in CC cycle is not of much benefit.
- Progesterone support is required in letrozole-stimulated cycle.
- Dydrogesterone and SR tablets are under trial.
- All superovulated cycles require luteal support.
- Agonist and antagonist cycles cause LPD.
- With GnRHa trigger, luteal support is always required.
- Judicious use of E2 + P, dual trigger or 1,500 IU of hCG at the time can be used for luteal support.
- E2 supplementation is given for LPS in agonist trigger.
- Endometriosis and PCOS have progesterone resistance.
- Duration of progesterone after positive beta-hCG is controversial.

REFERENCES

1. Hill MJ, Whitcomb B, Lewis TD, Wu M, Terry N, DeCherney AH, et al. Progesterone as luteal support after ovulation induction and IUI: a systematic review and meta-analysis. Fertil Steril. 2013;100(5):1373-80.
2. Speroff L, Fritz MA. Clinical Gynecologic Endocrinology and Infertility, 7th re-edition. Philadelphia: Lippincott Williams and Wilkins; 2005. pp. 199-242.
3. Kyrou D, Fatemi HM, Tournaye H, Devroey P. Luteal phase support in normo-ovulatory women stimulated with clomiphene citrate for intrauterine insemination: need or habit? Hum Reprod. 2010;25(10):2501-6.
4. Dickey RP. Evaluation and management of threatened and habitful first trimester abortion. In: Osofsky H (Ed). Advances in Clinical Obstetrics and Gynecology, Volume 2. Chicago: Yearbook Medical Publishers; 1984. pp. 329-88.
5. Montville CP, Khabba M, Aubuchon M, Williams DB, Thomas MA. Luteal support with intravaginal progesterone increases clinical pregnancy rates in women with polycystic ovary syndrome using letrozole for ovulation induction. Fertil Steril. 2010;94(2):678-83.
6. Tavaniotou A, Albano C, Smitz J, Devroey P. Impact of ovarian stimulation on corpus luteum function and embryonic implantation. J Reprod Immunol. 2002;55(1-2):123-30.
7. Xu B, Li Z, Zhang H, Jin L, Li Y, Ai J, et al. Serum progesterone level effects on the outcome of in vitro fertilization in patients with different ovarian response: an analysis of more than 10,000 cycles. Fertil Steril. 2012;97(6):1321-7.
8. Doldi N, Marsiglio E, Destefanu A, Gessi A, Merati G, Ferrari A. Elevated serum P on the day of hCG administration in IVF is associated with a higher pregnancy rate in polycystic ovary syndrome. Hum Reprod. 1999;14(3):1601-5.
9. Humaidan P, Ejdrup Bredkjaer H, Westergard LG, Andersen CY. 1,500 IU human chorionic gonadotropins administered at oocyte retrieval rescues the luteal phase when gonadotropin-releasing hormone agonist is used for ovulation induction: a prospective, randomized, controlled study. Fertil Steril. 2010;93(3):847-54.

10. Fatemi HM. The luteal phase after 3 decades of IVF: what do we know? Reprod Biomed Online. 2009;19 Suppl 4:4331.
11. Devroey P, Bourgain C, Macklon NS, Fauser BCJM. Reproductive biology and IVF: ovarian stimulation and endometrial receptivity. Trends Endocrinol Metab. 2004;15(2): 84-90.
12. Humaidan P, Papnikolaou EG, Kyrou D, Alsbjerg B, Polyzos NP, Devroey P, et al. The luteal phase after GnRH agonist triggering of ovulation: present and future perspectives. Reprod Biomed Online. 2012;24(2): 134-41.
13. Miyake A, Aono T, Kinugasa T, Tanizawa O, Kurachi K. Suppression of serum levels of luteinizing hormone by short and long-loop negative feedback in ovariectomized women. J Endocrinol. 1979;80(3):353-6.
14. Vander Linden H, Buckingham K, Farquhar C, Kremer JA, Metwally M. Luteal support for assisted reproduction cycles. Cochrane Database Syst rev. 2011;(10):CD009154.
15. Cantineau AE, Cohlen BJ, Heineman MJ. Ovarian stimulation protocols (antioestrogens, gonadotrophins with and without GnRH agonists/antagonists) for intrauterine insemination (IUI) in women with subfertility. Cochrane Database Syst Rev. 2007;(18): CD005356.
16. Panchal S, Nagori CB. Ultrasound based decision making on stimulation protocols for superovulated IUI cycles. IJIFM. 2016;7(1): 7-13.
17. Papanikolaou EG, Verpoest W, Fatemi H, Tarlatzis B, Devroey P, Tournaye H. A novel method of luteal supplementation with recombinant luteinizing hormone when a gonadotropin releasing hormone agonist issued instead of human chorionic gonadotropin for ovulation trigger: a randomized prospective proof of concept study. Fertil Steril. 2011;95(3):1174-7.
18. Fatemi HM, Kolibianakis EM, Camus M, Tournaye H, Donoso P, Papanikolaou E, et al. Addition of estradiol to progesterone for luteal supplementation in patients stimulated with GnRH antagonists/rFSH for IVF: a randomized controlled trial. Hum Reprod. 2006;21(10):2628-32.
19. Anderson CY, Elbaek HO, Alsbjerg B, Laursen RJ, Povisen BB, Thomsen L, et al. Daily low-dose hCG stimulation during the luteal phase combined with GnRHa triggered IVF cycles without exogenous progesterone: a proof of concept trial. Hum Reprod. 2015; 30(10):2387-95.
20. Erdem A, Erdem M, Atmaca S, Guler I. Impact of luteal phase support on pregnancy rates in intrauterine insemination cycles: A prospective randomized study. Fertil Steril. 2009;91(6):2508-13.
21. Maher MA. Luteal phase support may improve pregnancy outcomes during intrauterine insemination cycles. Eur J Obstet Gynecol Reprod Biol. 2011;157(1):57-62.
22. Tavaniotou A, Devroey P. Effect of human chorionic gonadotropins on luteal luteinizing hormone concentrations in natural cycles. Fertil Steril. 2003;80(3):654-5.
23. Kummer N, Benadiva C, Feinn R, Mann J, Nulsen J, Engmann L. Factors that predict the probability of successful clinical outcome after induction of oocyte maturation with gonadotropin-releasing hormone agonist. Fertil Steril. 2011;96(1):63-8.
24. Evans J, Salamonsen LA. Too much of a good thing? Experimental evidence suggests prolonged exposure to hCG is detrimental to endometrial receptivity. Hum Reprod. 2013;28(6):1610-9.
25. Anderson Y, Fisher R, Giorgione V, Kelsey TW. Microdose hCG as luteal support without exogenous progesterone administration. Mathematical model of hCG concentration in circulation and initial experience. J Assist Reprod Genet. 2016;33(10):1311-8.
26. Nyboe AA, Popovic-Todorovic B, Schmidt KT, Loft A, Lindhard A, Højgaard A, et al. Progesterone supplementation during early gestations after IVF and ICSI has no effect on the delivery rates: a randomized controlled trial. Hum Reprod. 2002;17(2):357-61.
27. Caspo AI, Pulkkinen MO, Wiest WG. Effects of lutectomy and progesterone replacement therapy in early pregnant patients. Am J Obstet Gynecol. 1973;115(6):759-65.
28. Schmidt KL, Ziebe S, Popovic B, Lindhard A, Loft A, Andersen AN. Progesterone supplementation during early gestation after in vitro fertilization has no effect on delivery rate. Fertil Steril. 2001;75(2):337-41.
29. Mochtar MH, Van Wely M, Van der Veen F. Timing luteal phase support in GnRH agonist downregulated IVF/embryo transfer cycles. Hum Reprod. 2006;21(4):905-8.

CHAPTER 10

Complications of Intrauterine Insemination

INTRODUCTION

This discussion will be divided into:

- *Complications related to stimulation protocol:*
    - Ovarian hyperstimulation syndrome (OHSS)
    - Multiple pregnancy
- *Complications related to procedure:*
    - Infection

COMPLICATIONS RELATED TO STIMULATION PROTOCOL

Ovarian Hyperstimulation Syndrome

Regular obstetricians and gynecologists are afraid of giving gonadotropins as they fear OHSS. But OHSS is not common in intrauterine insemination (IUI) cycles. It can occur in PCOS patients or hyper-responders only. If the baseline score[1] with dose chart is used, risk of OHSS can be almost absolutely eliminated. Chronic low-dose protocol is the usual gonadotropin regime for these patients.

When higher doses are given, or sometimes in spite of chronic low-dose protocol, multiple follicles may develop. If apart from mature follicles of 16–18 mm or larger, there are 4–5 follicles of 11–14 mm in both the ovaries, human chorionic gonadotropin (hCG) should not be given as a trigger. Instead gonadotropin-releasing hormone (GnRH) agonist is given. GnRHa causes luteal phase defect, but this can be corrected by:

- E2 + P in luteal phase
- 1,500 IU of hCG as a single shot after IUI

These treatment regimens are discussed in detail in the chapter on luteal phase support.

Suppose hCG is already given as a trigger, OHSS can be prevented by:

- Tablet Cabergoline 0.5 mg for 8 days
- Hydroxyethyl starch (HES) (starch) can be given at the time of IUI.

Some practitioners convert IUI cycle into in vitro fertilization (IVF) cycle, but this is not required. We have never done that. Ultrasound can predict OHSS and if estradiol level is also >1600 IU on the day of trigger, do not give hCG as a trigger. We rely more on ultrasound, rather than estradiol levels. If there are more than 3–4 follicles of between the diameter of 11 and 14 mm, on both the sides, hCG trigger is not given.

Ovarian hyperstimulation syndrome can occur even if a patient had developed multiple follicles and GnRHa trigger is given, if patient conceives in that cycle. But it is usually mild to moderate and can be treated conservatively.

Multiple Pregnancy

Gonadotropin with IUI gives higher pregnancy rate at the cost of the risk of multiple pregnancies. It is reported as high as 11.7% twin pregnancy rate and 0.5% triplet pregnancies.[2]

Identification of Risk Factors

Pregnancy rate reported with monofollicular development was 8.4% as compared to 15% for multifollicular development.[3] In the same study, the risk of multiple pregnancy rate after 2, 3, and 4 follicles was 6, 14, and 10%. So, our aim should be to get 2–3 follicles after stimulation, as higher number of follicles do not increase pregnancy rate. The number of follicles must be adjusted to woman's age to limit the risk of multiple pregnancies as shown by the absence of multiple pregnancies in women older than 38 years even with three follicles and the high multiple pregnancy rate 38% in younger than 28 years even with two follicles. Antagonist helps after 28 years for better pregnancy rate.[4]

Stimulation Protocol

Cochrane review has confirmed that gonadotropin has higher pregnancy rate than antiestrogens without increasing multiple pregnancy rate. Doubling the gonadotropin dose in IUI does not increase pregnancy rate.[5] But, multiple pregnancy rate is always dependent on number of follicles rather than type of product. Dosing according to nomogram is superior to standard dosing.[3]

We always calculate the ovulation induction dose from our baseline score,[1] which gives high pregnancy rate with low multiple pregnancy rate and very low high-order multiple pregnancy.

Multiple pregnancy may lead to maternal complications such as diabetes, pregnancy-induced hypertension (PIH), operative delivery, and postpartum hemorrhage (PPH), and fetal complications such as respiratory distress syndrome, intraventricular hemorrhage, and pneumonia may occur due to prematurity. Late complications such as growth restriction, cerebral palsy, mental retardation, and limited motor and cognitive skill deformity may occur due to prematurity.

When more than 15 follicles of >7 mm are present at the start of stimulation, high-order multiple follicles may develop. But, in today's era, such stimulation is never given for IUI patients. Chronic low-dose protocol avoids high order multiple pregnancy.

Follicles larger than 10 mm, especially those larger than or equal to 12 mm may need to be clearly recorded during transvaginal ultrasound surveillance and their potential effects on both pregnancy and multiple pregnancy can be discussed with couples undergoing IUI. In a study of 13000 cycles, the author found a high incidence of multiple pregnancy in IUI with more 12–14 mm sized follicles.[6]

Secondary Preventive Measures

- *Cancellation of cycle:* We have never come across this situation, as the stimulation protocol should be according to the baseline score.[1] Professor Roy Homburg has also found lower OHSS and multiple pregnancy rate with chronic low-dose protocol. So, it is important to always give a rethought before starting stimulation for a PCOS patient.[7] With availability of antagonist protocol with agonist trigger, OHSS and multiple pregnancy rate can be decreased.
- *Aspiration of supernumerary follicles:* It is an invasive procedure. On the day of trigger, ultrasound-guided aspiration is done when there are more than 4 follicles developed. It can reduce multiple pregnancy rate to 0–10%.[5]

  We have never done this procedure and have never heard of centers in India doing this practice for IUI.
- *Escape IVF:* Convert IUI cycle into IVF cycle. This is never required, if your stimulation protocol is precise. Patients will not be ready for spending exorbitant amount for the procedure. On the top of it, as there are multiple follicles, you will freeze the embryos for the fear of OHSS.

  In my opinion, therefore, to convert IUI to IVF is an iatrogenic complication. I have never done in my practice. Starting dose of stimulation is much more important. It should be according to the baseline score system.[1]

Antagonists cannot be used always to prevent premature LH surge because when the decision is taken, size of the follicle may be >14 mm and then antagonist may or may not prevent the LH surge.

- *Selective reduction:* This can be done by the experts. If there is high-order multiple pregnancy, it should be reduced to twins. It is less costly as compared to converting IUI into IVF cycle. But it has a risk of abortion due to the procedure.

COMPLICATIONS RELATED TO PROCEDURE

Infection

- Patient evaluation and screening
- Sperm preparation to reduce infection
- Environmental and procedural contamination

Patient Evaluation

Do viral testing, as these can be transmitted through semen and vaginal secretion, e.g., cytomegalovirus (CMV), hepatitis B virus (HBV), hepatitis C virus (HCV), hepatitis D virus (HDV), herpes simplex virus (HSV)-2 and human immunodeficiency virus (HIV), etc. So, all biological samples should be handled carefully. Semen culture in asymptomatic patient is not required. Microbes are present in 50% of all semen samples obtained by masturbation. So, strict guidelines are given for collection. Antibiotics according to infections can be prescribed. Nonspermicidal condom is preferred over coitus interruptus for semen collection. Treat both patients before IUI.

Sperm Preparation

- Sterile disposables are to be used.
- Density-gradient method is to be used.
- Media should be properly stored as per instructions.
- For HIV-positive male, IUI with washed sample is the only option.

Environmental and Procedural Aspect

- Good laboratory facilities and disposables
- Cross-contamination should be prevented.
- Proper identification of samples
- Eating, drinking, and smoking are prohibited in the laboratory. Staff entry is to be restricted. Unhygienic working conditions and waste disposal definitely increased risk of infection transmission to personnel, patients, cultures, samples, and equipment.

The practical aspect is that patients may get moderate or severe pain after few minutes to few hours after IUI. This pain may be due to foreign material introduced or infection because of contaminated sample. The disadvantage is that there is a severe uterine spasm and the patient does not conceive in that cycle. Moreover, patient develops avulsion for the procedure. It is therefore important that the semen is prepared with all due precautions and in sterile conditions. The media needs to be checked for any contamination from time to time and if contaminated, it needs to be discarded. Disposables should be checked for their sterility. Any pain after IUI should be taken seriously and antispasmodics should be given to relieve it, and antibiotics may be given to treat the infection.

CARRY HOME MESSAGE

- OHSS can be prevented by chronic low-dose protocol or lower dose according to the baseline score.
- Cabergoline and HES can be used as preventive measures.
- Conversion of IUI into IVF is very costly and can be prevented.
- Multiple pregnancy can be prevented by lower doses.
- Full aseptic precautions should be taken during preparation of sample.

REFERENCES

1. Panchal S, Nagori CB. Ultrasound based decision making on stimulation protocols for superovulated IUI cycles. IJIFM. 2016;7(1): 7-13.
2. de Mouzon J, Goossens V, Bhattacharya S, Castilla JA, Ferraretti AP, Korsak V, et al. Assisted Reproductive technology in Europe, 2007: Results generated from European registers by ESHRE. Hum Reprod. 2012;27(4): 954-66.
3. Van Rumste MM, Custers IM, Van der Veen F, Van Wely M, Evers JL, Mol BW. The influence of number of follicles on pregnancy rate in intrauterine insemination with ovarian stimulation: a meta-analysis. Hum Reprod Update. 2008;14(6):563-70.
4. Monrasion O, Chansel-Debordeaux L, Chiron A, Floret S, Cens S, Bourrinet S, et al. Evaluation of intrauterine insemination practice: a 1-year prospective study in seven French assisted reproduction technology centers. Fertil Steril. 2016;105(6):1589-93.
5. Cantineau AE, Cohlen BJ, Heineman MJ. Ovarian stimulation protocols (antioestrogens, gonadotrophins with and without GnRH agonists/antagonists) for intrauterine insemination (IUI) in women with subfertility. Cochrane Database Syst Rev. 2007;(2): CD005356.
6. Du T, Xie Q, Qiu J, Zhang S, Mol BW, Kuang Y, Zhao D, Li W. Effect of small follicles on clinical pregnancy and multiple pregnancy rates in intrauterine insemination: a cohort study. Hum Reprod. 2024;39(2):335-45.
7. Mc Clamrock HD, Jones HW Jr, Adashi EY. Ovarian stimulation and intrauterine insemination at the quarter centennial: implications for the multiple births epidemic. Fertil Steril. 2012;97(4):802-9.

CHAPTER 11

Factors Affecting Intrauterine Insemination Success

INTRODUCTION

Success of intrauterine insemination (IUI) is dependent on several variables. Some of these are already discussed at other places in this book and the rest are discussed here:

- Female age
- Male age
- Weight of the patient
- Time interval
- Serum progesterone on day of the trigger

FEMALE AGE

There is a gradual decline in monthly fecundity after 30 years and sharp decrease after 35 years of female age. It is documented that natural fertility ends at 41 years. In human being, monthly fecundity is only 20%, so it is low fertility and, therefore, human beings require several months to conceive. The incidence of infertility in females in their 20s is only 4%, it is 10–20% till 35 years then, and reaches about 50% after 35 years. These patients usually have a long-term infertility. Beyond 35 years, the quality of the ova also deteriorates and incidence of aneuploidies in the fetuses increases.

The recommendations are that in a couple with unexplained infertility, IUI should be limited to couples with female age under 40 years. No routine ovarian reserve screening prior to starting IUI treatment is required. IUI may be advised with donor sperm for up to 42 years. Ovarian reserve testing is required only to exclude older women and for them, effective treatment is only ovum donation. So, ovarian reserve tests are not required in IUI practice.[1] In women aged ≤38 years, IUI should be considered as an option particularly in cases of female factor infertility due to ovulatory disorder, in cases of normal ovarian reserve, in cases of secondary infertility, or when postwash semen count in a male is ≥1 million with progressive motility >90%. In all these cases, bifollicular development with ovulation induction improves the chance of pregnancy.[2]

Young patients of <35 years of age with diminished ovarian reserve (AMH <1.0 ng/mL) conceived as often and had pregnancy outcome similar to those of age-matched controls (AMH ≥1.0 ng/mL) after IUI. Only higher dose of FSH is required for similar outcome. Cumulative conceptions and live-birth rates were also similar in young patients with normal and diminished ovarian reserve.[3]

MALE AGE

Advanced male age is associated with a decline in semen volume, sperm motility, and morphology but not with sperm concentration. These parameters start declining after 35 years. DNA damage at older age may give multiple genetic and chromosomal defects. After 40 years, it has negative effect on IUI success rate. But, there is no absolute cut off for the age as far as male infertility is concerned.

There are few reports that as paternal age advances, pregnancy rates are lower, but it has influence only when female age is also >35 years. Paternal age has no impact on IUI success rate as long as female partner's age is <35 years. Synergistic effect of paternal age only exists when female partner is >35 years of age.[4] Though it may increase miscarriage rates.[5,6] Miscarriage rate is increased, if paternal age is more because of oxidative stress-induced mtDNA damage and nuclear DNA damage. This damage may put them at a higher risk of transmitting multiple genetic and chromosomal defects.

INFLUENCE OF WEIGHT

Female obesity is associated with lower oocyte yield with gonadotropin stimulation, lower pregnancy rate, and increased pregnancy loss in IVF (in vitro fertilization).[7] But, fecundity rates are higher in obese patients particularly in polycystic ovary syndrome (PCOS). Weight loss improves obstetric outcome and not fecundity. The optimal body mass index (BMI) for natural fecundity may be between 20 and 24. Detailed studies are not available on obesity and fertility. So, BMI has proven to be a practical indicator of obesity.

In patients undergoing gonadotropin-IUI treatment, miscarriage rates are not significantly higher in obese patients compared to women with normal BMI. In women undergoing IUI treatment, BMI guidelines used for IVF cannot be applied.

TIME INTERVAL FOR INTRAUTERINE INSEMINATION

There is no randomized study on this topic. Semen sample should be delivered within 1 hour of collection, spermatozoa survive for 12–24 hours, and acceptable motility is found up to 12 hours. Though spermatozoa will survive for 24–48 hours after semen preparation.

COLLECTION INSEMINATION TIME

Optimum is approximately 80–120 minutes without significant difference.[8]

- *Collection preparation interval:* If this is between 20 and 40 minutes, the results are better.[9]
- *Preparation instrumentation interval:* It is between 10 and 40 minutes for those who become pregnant.[8] So still, ample research is required for time intervals. But, reduced time interval is recommended for good pregnancy rate. Especially, interval between collection and processing should be less than 1 hour preferably 45 minutes.

During IUI treatment, wildfire smoke has a negative impact as it lowers total motile count (TMC).[10]

SERUM PROGESTERONE ON THE DAY OF TRIGGER

When progesterone is elevated on the day of ovulation trigger, counseling should be done with patients that IUI may give lesser success rate and timing of insemination should be managed to optimize implantation.[11] Whenever progesterone rise occurs, trigger is given earlier to improve the IUI results. In chronic low-dose protocol in PCOS, it is extremely rare to get progesterone rise. It is more common in IVF rather than IUI.

Live-birth rates are higher when progesterone ranges from 1.0 to 1.5 ng/mL, rather than higher or lower. It may be prognostic indicator for OS-IUI.[12] Higher progesterone >1.5 ng/mL may cause endometrial asynchrony and reduced pregnancy rates in ART. But in IUI, there is mild ovarian stimulation, so there is not much premature progesterone rise.

High progesterone and high estrogen are found in clomiphene citrate cycle but not with letrozole. The relationship between estradiol and progesterone is found in gonadotropin stimulated cycles where higher estradiol is frequently observed which gives higher pregnancy rate.

LH surge is noted in 30% of CC cycles and 42% of gonadotropin cycles. So higher pregnancy rate was observed when there was no LH surge.[13]

The rise in progesterone is responsible for true trigger of midcycle LH surge and it helps in function of corpus luteum. So high progesterone indicates ovulation induction and IUI, may be late and conception rate after intercourse is also possible as oocyte is in the fallopian tube. Even IUI, shortly after ovulation can also give pregnancy.

Semen wash count: Study of 9347 cycles by Muthigi et al. showed that the IUI pregnancy rates were optimal with total motile sperm count (TMSC) of >9 × 10^6, below which pregnancy rate declines. Although rare pregnancies were achieved even with TMSC of 0.25 × 10^6. Since the decline is gradual and continuous, there is no specific threshold above which IUI should be recommended. These more quantitative predictors can be used to provide personalized counseling and guide clinical decision making.[14] In those with low TMSC, pooling of the semen sample can be done and that can reduce the number of treatment cycles.

It has also been documented that with increasing age of female partner, clinical pregnancy rate for given TMSC is lower compared to the cohort of younger women. Naturally, therefore for a given TMSC, couples with younger women have better clinical pregnancy rate. Couples with younger women may have a better clinical pregnancy rate even with lower TMSC. At an age of 41–42 years, the conception rate with IUI is 5–8% and that with IVF is 9%. Therefore, in such cases other associated factors should be considered to decide on the trial for number of IUI cycles.

It must be kept in mind that the factors that affect the pregnancy rate with IUI also include:[15]

1. Discomfort during procedure—decreases pregnancy rate.
2. Time from trigger to IUI

And on the other hand, it also must be kept in mind that bleeding during procedure and type of catheter have no impact on pregnancy rate and TMSC of upto 5 × 10^6, has same pregnancy rate.

CARRY HOME MESSAGE

- Age is the single factor that decreases fecundability.
- IUI must be tried before 38–40 years of age.
- Age of the male partner is not of much importance for pregnancy.
- Obesity is more related to obstetric outcomes rather than infertility.
- Semen collection to insemination time should be 80–120 minutes.
- Progesterone on the day of trigger is not required for improving IUI results.

REFERENCES

1. Broekmans FJ, Soules MR, Fauser BC. Ovarian aging: mechanisms and clinical consequences. Endocr Rev. 2009;30(5):465-93.
2. Dinelli L, Courbiere B, Achard V, Jouve E, Deveze C, Gnisci A, et al. Prognosis factors of pregnancy after intrauterine insemination with husband's sperm: conclusion of an analysis of 2019 cycles. Fertil Steril. 2014;101(4):994-1000.
3. Tiegs AW, Sun L, ScottJr RT, Goodman LR. Comparison of pregnancy outcomes following intrauterine insemination in young women with decreased versus normal ovarian reserve. Fertil Steril. 2020;113(4):788-95.
4. Brzechffa PR, Buyalos RP. Female and male partner age and menotrophin requirements influence pregnancy rates with human menopausal gonadotrophin therapy in combination with intrauterine insemination. Hum Reprod. 1997;12(1):29-33.
5. Mathieu C, Ecochard R, Bied V, Lornage J, Czyba JC. Cumulative conception rate following intrauterine artificial insemination with husband's spermatozoa: influence of husband's age. Hum Reprod. 1995;10(5): 1090-7.

6. de La Rochebrochard E, Thonneau P. Paternal age and maternal age are risk factors for miscarriage: results of a multicentre European study. Hum Reprod. 2002;17(6):1649-56.
7. Fedorcsák P, Dale PO, Storeng R, Ertzeid G, Bjercke S, Oldereid N, et al. Impact of overweight and underweight on assisted reproduction treatment. Hum Reprod. 2004;19(11):2523-8.
8. Yavas Y, Selub MR. Intrauterine insemination (IUI) pregnancy outcome is enhanced by shorter interval from semen collection to sperm wash, from sperm wash to IUI time, and from semen collection to IUI time. Fertil Steril. 2004;82(6):1638-47.
9. Ramón O, Corcostegui B, Crisol L, Exposito A, Mugica J, Matorras R. Sperm processing: The time interval as prognostic factor in intrauterine insemination (IUI). 27th Annual meeting of the ESHRE. Stockholm, Sweden July 3-7, 2011. Hum Reprod. 2011;26(Suppl 1):i112.
10. Rubin ES, Kornfield M, Parker P, Garg B, O'leary T, Baldwin M, Krieg S. Poor quality air from wild fire smoke is associated with decrease in total motile count at time of intrauterine insemination. Fertil Steril. 2024;121(5):881-3.
11. Requena A, Cruz M, Pacheco A, Gracia-Valesco JA. Ongoing pregnancy rates in IUI are affected by late follicular phase progesterone levels. Fertil Steril. 2015;104(4):879-83.
12. Burks HR, Peck JD, Gavrizi S, Anderson ZS, Diamond MP, Hansen KR. Effect of prematurely elevated late follicular progesterone on pregnancy outcome following ovarian stimulation-intrauterine insemination for unexplained infertility: secondary analysis of the AMIGOS trial. Hum Reprod. 2024; 39(8):1684-91.
13. Cantineau AE, Janssen MJ, Cohlen bj, Allersma T. Synchronized approach for intrauterine insemination in subfertile couples. Cochrane Database Syst Rev. 2014;(12):CD006942.
14. Muthigi A, Jahandideh S, Bishop LA, Naemmi FK, Shipley SK, O'Brein JE, et al. Clarifying the relationship between total mobile sperm counts and intrauterine insemination pregnancy rates. Fertil Steril. 2021;115:1454-60.
15. Hansen KR, Peck JD, Coward RM, Wild RA, Trussell JC, Krawetz SA, et al. Intrauterine insemination performance characteristics and post-processing total motile sperm count in relation to live birth for couples with unexplained infertility in a randomised, multicentre clinical trial. Hum Reprod. 2020; 35(6):1296-305.

CHAPTER

12

Sperm Preparation

INTRODUCTION

After assessment of the semen sample, preparation is done. The preparation of the semen sample depends on the count, motile sperms, volume, viscosity, and presence of antibodies, white blood cell (WBC), and debris.

The purpose of semen preparation is to concentrate the normal motile sperms with intact functional and genetic properties including normal morphology, minimal DNA damage, and intact cell membranes with functional binding properties. It makes sperms hyperactive after removal of seminal plasma **(Fig. 1)**. Seminal plasma has prostaglandins, anticapacitation and antifertilization factors, dead sperms, WBC, bacteria, and germ cells.

Proteins and buffers in media promote sperm capacitation, while serum appears to be important for sperm motility. Inclusion of protein is required to prevent sperm adhering to surfaces. Bicarbonate is required for capacitation. Media-containing glucose is always better.

COLLECTION OF SEMEN SAMPLE

Abstinence is not preferred before intrauterine insemination (IUI), as long abstinence may result in higher sperm volume and concentration, but results in lower sperm motility and high sperm DNA fragmentation levels. Though 24 hours of abstinence is advised, as abstinence shorter than that may result in poor chromatin packaging. It has been shown that IUI outcomes were optimal after 2 days of ejaculatory abstinence[1] and, therefore, ≤2 days of abstinence is advised before IUI.

It is collected by aseptic technique in sterilized jar **(Fig. 2)**. Water or wet hands must not touch semen or the inner surface

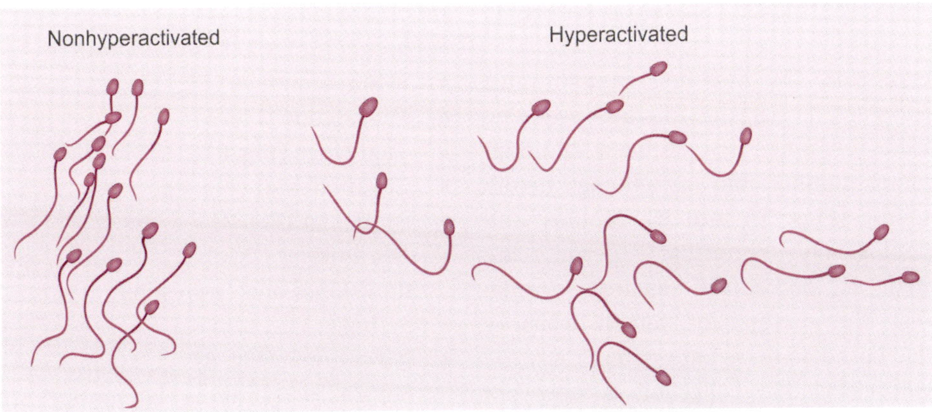

Fig. 1: Diagrammatic presentation of nonhyperactivated sperms in semen sample and hyperactivated sperms in processed semen sample.

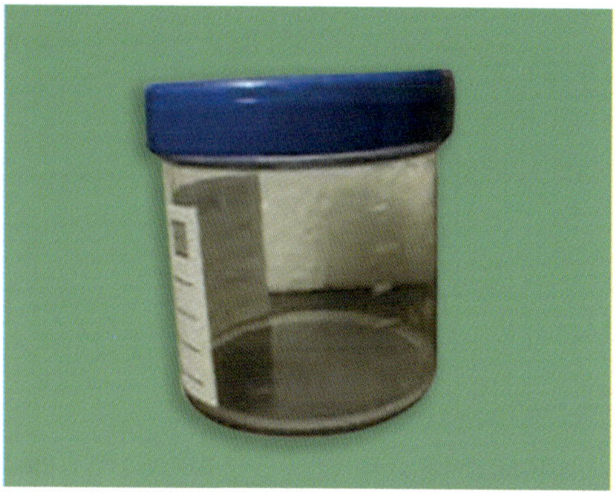

Fig. 2: Ethylene oxide (ETO) sterilized semen collection jar.

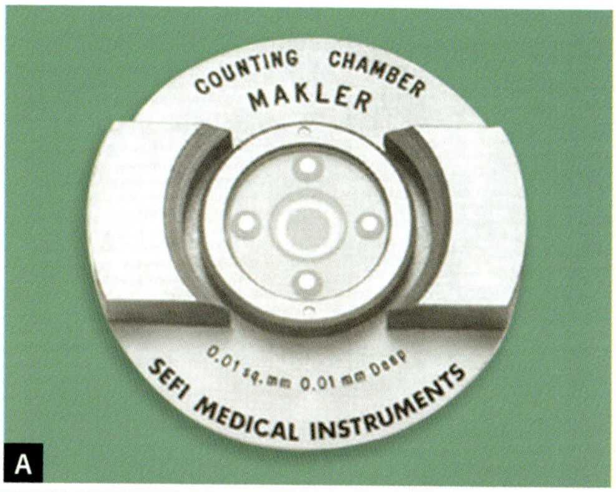

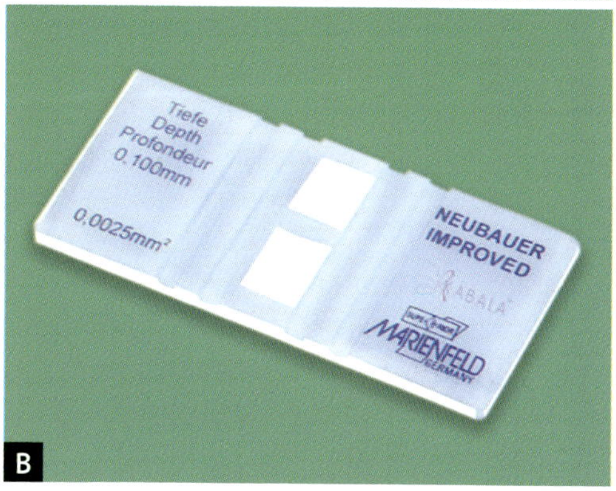

Figs. 3A and B: (A) Makler's chamber; (B) Neubar's chamber.

of the jar. Ask the patient to clean and dry parts before collection. Possibly, collection should be done in the premises, but if not the case, transport time from collection to incubator should not be >30 minutes at body temperature. Seminal plasma contains several substances that may reduce the fertilizing capacity of the sperms.[2] During transport, semen should not be exposed to direct sunlight.

Semen is allowed to stand in the incubator at 37°C temperature for liquefaction for 20–30 minutes. Semen preparation should begin as soon as possible after liquefaction. Liquefaction is required for homogeneous population of sperms throughout the semen sample. If liquefaction does not occur, needling through 23-gauge needle can be done, though sperm damage is known to occur by this.

As a rule, the liquefied sample must be examined under the microscope using Meckler's chamber or Neubar's chamber for count, motility, and morphology before processing **(Figs. 3A and B)**. Motility and morphologically abnormal sperms are counted as percentage against normal sperms. The method of semen wash is decided based on these parameters.

Split ejaculation collection is now not recommended, as the results are the same and spillage can occur with split ejaculation.

When antisperm antibodies are present, semen is collected directly in culture media, as it decreases free antibodies and improves chances of fertilization. Similarly, semen with high viscosity is also collected in culture media.

Instruments and equipment required for good sperm preparation:

- Incubator for 37°C temperature
- Laminar air flow **(Fig. 4)**
- Microscope **(Fig. 5)**
- Centrifuge **(Fig. 6)**
- CO_2 incubator **(Fig. 7)**
- Semen jar **(Fig. 2)**
- *Disposables:* Double lock tubes, pipette, tips, slides, and cover slips
- Syringe
- IUI cannula **(Fig. 8)**

Sperm preparation laboratory should preferably be in the same set-up where IUI is to be done. Laboratory should be a cool

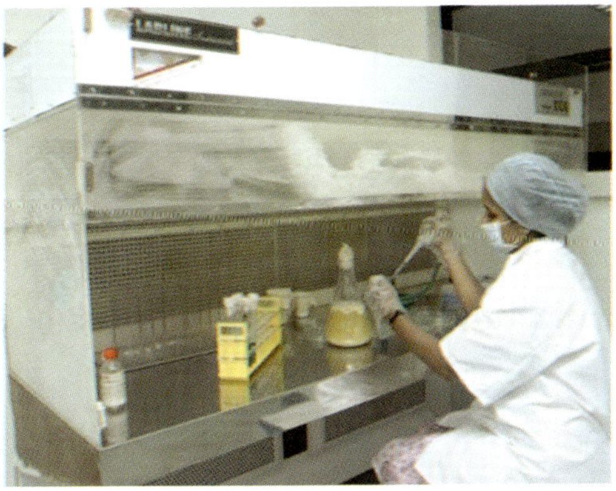

Fig. 4: Laminar air flow.

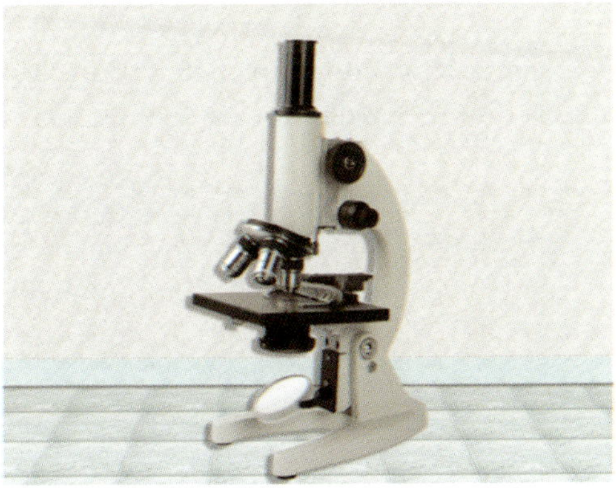

Fig. 5: Microscope.

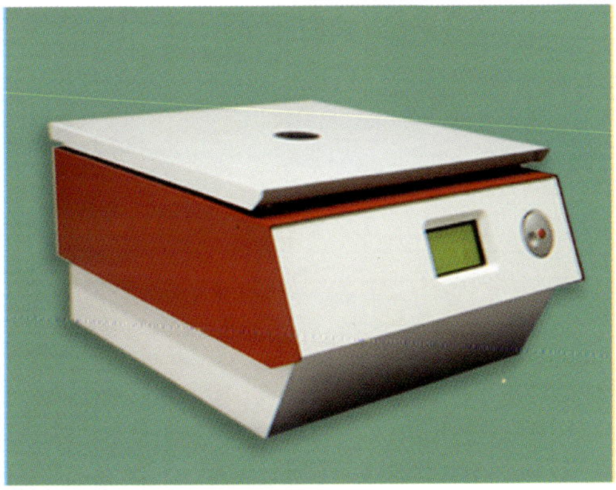

Fig. 6: Centrifuge machine.

place and should not have windows and should not be in the direction of sunlight for long hours of the day. It should preferably not be the top floor of the building.

Composition of sperm preparation media:
- Earle's balance media
- Sodium pyruvate as antioxidant
- Synthetic serum replacement
- HEPES buffer for maintaining pH
- Sodium bicarbonate for capacitation
- Human serum albumin 1% for capacitation, prevents sperm adhering and motility
- Penicillin 50,000 IU/L + streptomycin 50 mg/L to prevent bacterial contamination
- Phenol red
- Glucose for energy

Selection of method depends on:
- Motile count
- Volume of semen
- Presence of leukocytes, debris, and other cells
- Viscosity

Whether it is for IUI, in vitro fertilization (IVF), or intracytoplasmic sperm injection (ICSI).

Normal semen parameters according to WHO guidelines, 2010[3] are given in **Table 1**.

SPERM PREPARATION METHODS

- Simple washing
- Swim up
- Density gradient method

Sperm preparation time of 40–80 minutes has a positive effect on pregnancy rate.[4]

Other methods such as migration gravity sedimentation and glass wool columns are rarely used now.

Simple Washing

It is the oldest method and is also known as simple dilution and washing technique. Only seminal plasma is removed by this technique; cellular debris, dead and nonmotile sperms, and bacteria are not removed completely, as there is no swim up. Semen is diluted with a large amount of medium (5–10 times of semen volume). It is then centrifuged at 300 g for 10 minutes with a purpose to wash it. Supernatant medium is removed, and pellet is resuspended in medium and

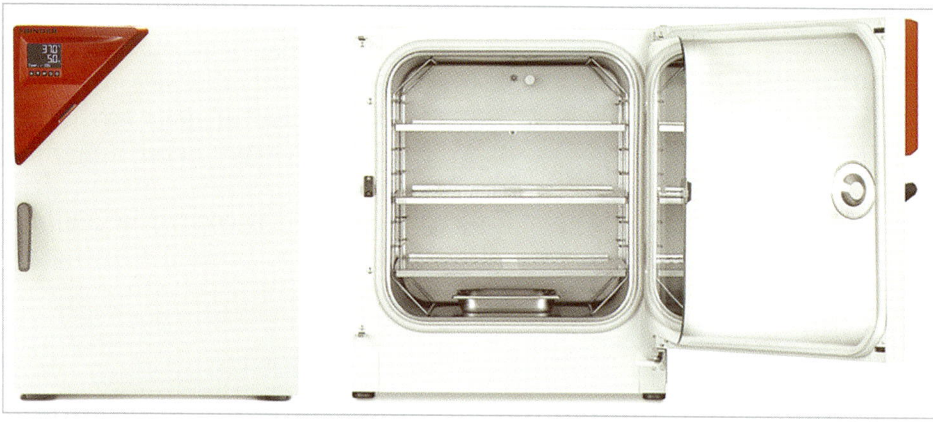

Fig. 7: Carbon dioxide (CO_2) incubator.

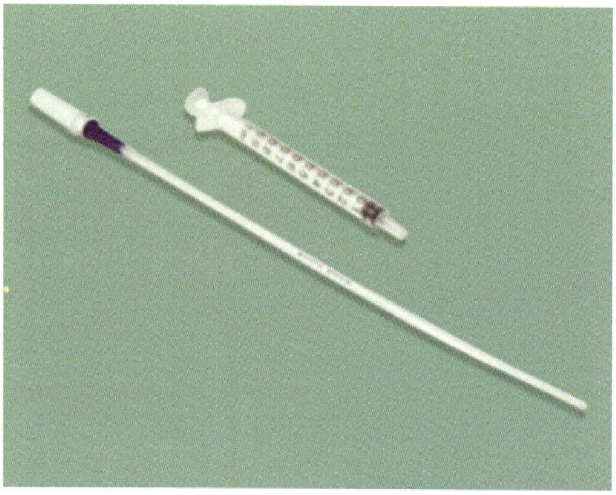

Fig. 8: Intrauterine insemination (IUI) cannula.

TABLE 1: Normal semen parameters according to World Health Organization (WHO) guidelines, 2010.

Seminal parameters	*Lower reference value*
Volume	1.5 mL
pH	7.2
Concentration	15 million/mL
Total number of sperms	39 million/ejaculate
Motility	40% total 32% progressive
Vitality	58% sperms alive/ ejaculate
Morphology	4% normal shape

again centrifuged at 300–500 g for 5 minutes. Again, the supernatant is removed, and the pellet is resuspended in medium appropriate for insemination and is incubated till insemination. This method is not used randomly.

Reagents for Swim up

- *Self-prepared medium:* Earle's balanced salt (EBSS) + streptopenicillin (penicillin 50,000 IU/L, streptomycin 50 mg/L + Na pyruvate + serum albumin
- *Readymade media* (available from various companies)
- Flushing medium, sperm preparation media (MediCult-Origio)
- Criopreparation (MediLine)
- G sperm (Scandinavian)
- FertiCult Flushing media

Swim-up Methods

- Swim up from ejaculate
- Swim up from pellet—different culture media have some variation **(Fig. 9)**

Swim up from ejaculate: This is the ideal method, as it does not require centrifugation.

- It is used only for normal semen sample.
- It is based on selection of the sperms based on their capability to swim up in the media.
- Morphologically abnormal sperms and reactive oxygen species (ROS) are not selected out.
- The total yield of sperms is lower than washing technique. It is therefore used for samples with high-sperm count.

Pellet—Swim up

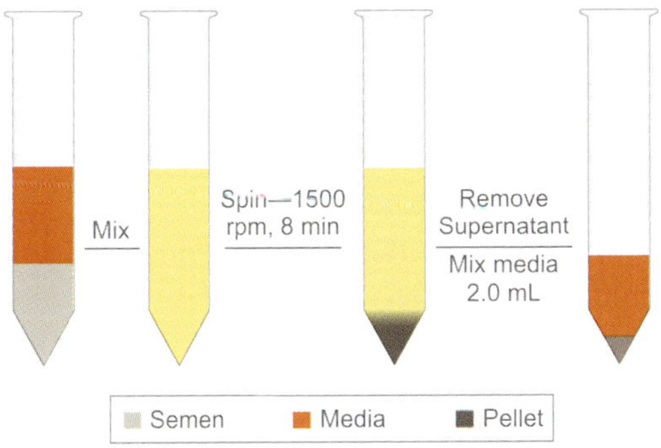

Fig. 9: Swim up from pellet.

- The time for which the samples are left for swim up depends on the total sperm count, but allowing to swim up for a long time allows more abnormal sperms to swim up.

Method: Aliquots of liquefied semen are placed directly under medium (1 mL) in round bottom tubes and these tubes are placed at 45° angle in a stand to be placed in the incubator for 30–60 minutes. The upper part of the layered medium from each test tube is collected, without disturbing the interface and washed in 2 mL medium by centrifuging at 300–500 g for 10 minutes. Then, the supernatant is removed, and pellet is resuspended in the amount of medium sufficient for insemination and incubated till insemination.

Swim up from pellet: This method is used for normal or marginally abnormal sperms, viscous samples, or samples collected in media.

Method: Take 2 mL of culture medium in a test tube:

- Pipette 1.5 mL of semen and mix it with medium
- Centrifuge at 300–500 g for 10 minutes
- Remove supernatant
- Resuspend the pellet in another 2 mL of medium
- Centrifuge for 5 minutes at 300 g
- Remove supernatant
- Layer the pellet with 1 mL of medium
- Put it in CO_2 incubator for swim up for 30–60 minutes
- Gently aspirate 0.5–0.7 mL of the solution from upper layers of medium, without disturbing the pellet.

Sperm capacitation requires the presence of bicarbonate ions. Therefore, if prepared sperms are stored before IUI, sperm buffer is advised, a zwitterions-buffered medium (such as HEPES). This will prevent premature capacitation and hyperactivated motility. If IUI is performed soon after sperm processing, bicarbonate buffered medium can be used for entire process.

This technique has the advantage of not using other chemicals than culture media. Most of the samples can be prepared by this method with different culture media. But alternative methods are also described. Flushing media is not commonly used for IUI swim up.

Method using sperm preparation media (swim up for sperms from ejaculate):

- Layer 1–1.5 mL of semen underneath 1–2 mL of pre-equilibrated sperm preparation media (SPM)
- The tubes are kept tilted in CO_2 incubator for 30–60 minutes.
- After swim up, upper 0.5–1 mL is aspirated and put it together.

Alternatively:

- Sample is diluted 1:3 v/v with media and is allowed to stand for 15 minutes at room temperature (+22°C).
- Centrifuge at 300 g for 10 minutes
- Remove supernatant and resuspend in 4 mL of SPM
- Centrifuge at 200 g for 5 minutes, remove supernatant
- Gently overlay the pellet with 2 mL of SPM and leave in CO_2 incubator for 120 minutes.
- Upper 0.1 mL has dead sperms and debris. This is removed.

- Then, the upper 0.7 mL is taken for insemination.

Variations: In non-ART centers, many gynecologists use flushing media rather than sperm preparation media. The difference in two media is given in **Table 2**.

To compensate for albumin content, add 5.62 mL of human albumin solution to 125 mL of bottle of flushing media. It gives equally good results with lower costs.

Swim up from pellet is most widely used method, as it separates motile sperms from nonmotile sperm and debris. Here, sperms are concentrated prior to swim up and do not have to escape seminal plasma. So, it is advantageous for viscous, moderate density, or moderate motility samples. It is suitable for samples collected in the media or cryopreserved samples.

The disadvantage of centrifuge is production of ROS, which is harmful for fertilization.

Method for sperm preparation media (MediCult):

- 2–4 test tubes with culture media are taken and in each tube, semen is put underneath the media. After 30 minutes, collect upper portion of each tube.
- Second alternative is that we can dilute semen three times with media and after 15 minutes centrifugation is done.
- First centrifugation is 300 g/10 min. Then resuspend in 4 mL of SPM.
- Then pellet is suspended with 2 mL in incubator for 60–120 minutes.

G sperm (Scandinavian media):

- Take 2–4 tubes with 1 mL semen

TABLE 2: Difference between flushing and sperm preparation media (SPM).

Component	*Flushing*	*SPM*
Albumin	0.1%	1.0%
pH	7–7.3	7.2–7.4
Bicarbonate	1.1	2.2

- Overlay with 2 mL media and incubate for 60 minutes
- Aspirate 1 mL from all tubes
- Add 5 mL media and centrifuge for 10 minutes at 300–600 g
- Discard supernatant

Repeat centrifugation after adding 5 mL media with 300–600 g for 10 minutes. Resuspend in G Fert and take 0.5–0.7 mL for insemination.

Tips for Better IUI

- Work under laminar airflow as far as possible and use completely sterile techniques.
- Gloves should not touch the inner side of the tubes; rubber is toxic for sperms.
- Work with more tubes rather than a single large tube when semen sample is large, or the count is too high.
- Leaving for swim up for a long time may allow the debris to swim up. Longer time may be required for swim up of low count or low motility samples that means an optimum time for swim up must be modified as per the count and motility of the sample.
- Semen processing is done within 30 minutes after collection and maximally within 1 hour.
- While loading, avoid contact of cannula with inner side of the tube.
- Rubber of syringe should not touch the sample that means when the sample is loaded in the cannula with the syringe attached, there should be a small air gap between the sample column and the rubber piston.
- Air should not be injected during IUI.
- No antiseptics are applied in the vagina.
- Equal volume of pentoxifylline solution can be added before centrifugation to improve motility in oligoasthenospermia.
- *For centrifuge machine:* Different companies have different parameters of

speed—the conversion formula is: rpm: $\sqrt{[g/(1.118 \times r)]}$

- Media is kept overnight in CO_2 incubator with loosened cap in a slanted test tube rack for equilibrium.
- With low count, large amount of semen may help.
- Clean the vagina and the vulva with normal saline before the wash, but it is not a must.
- Slanting test tube position during swim up allows larger surface and therefore larger sperm cohort **(Fig. 10)**.
- Proper labeling of tubes is a must.
- A good wash sample is one, which has at least 95% actively motile sperms and no debris.

Gradient Method

This is the method, which gives better recovery of sperms for IUI and conversion IVF. This method selects sperms according to their density and gravity (mass per unit volume) and results in cells being dispersed throughout the gradient column according to the gradient that matches their density. Normal spermatozoa have a density of 1.12 g/mL and immature abnormal sperms have density of 1.06 and 1.09 g/mL. Normal sperms can be isolated in the solution with highest concentration of gradient.

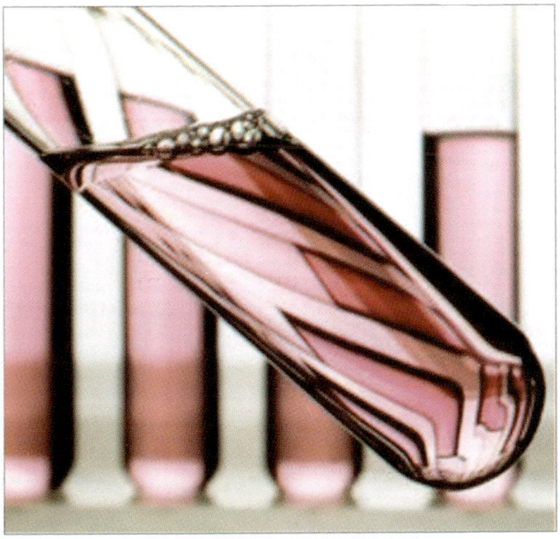

Fig. 10: Slanting position of the tube during swim up to allow better cohort of active sperms.

It is suitable for viscous samples as well as sample having more debris and WBCs and count is low. Dead and defective sperms and leukocytes produce ROS, which causes lipid peroxidation of sperm membrane and decreases motility. These are best removed by the gradient method. Debris and immotile sperms are held in-between gradient layers. Because of head density, sperms swim down and form pellet.

Some studies have shown that the method is more useful when percentage of sperms with progressive motility is lower and proportion of sperms with good morphology is lower. Higher centrifugation for shorter interval will give good recovery of motile sperms than when centrifugation is done at lower speed for longer time.

Different density gradient solutions are commercially available. But, we can make gradient media of 90% and 45%.

- Take 100% gradient media
- To make 90%, mix 0.9 mL of 100% gradient media and 0.1 mL of sperm preparation media.
- To make 45%, mix 0.45 mL of 100% gradient media and 0.55 mL of sperm preparation media.

Universal method **(Fig. 11)**:

- Layer 1 mL of 45% of density gradient media over 1 mL of 90% gradient media and above it, layer 1 mL of semen sample.
- Centrifuge at 1,500 rpm for 15 minutes.
- Remove supernatant.
- Transfer pellet to sterile centrifuge tube (may not be required).
- Add 3–5 mL of sperm preparation media and mix the pellet.
- Centrifuge at 1,000 rpm for 5 minutes.
- Remove supernatant.
- Mix pellet with 0.5–0.7 mL of washing media.
- Load the catheter for IUI.

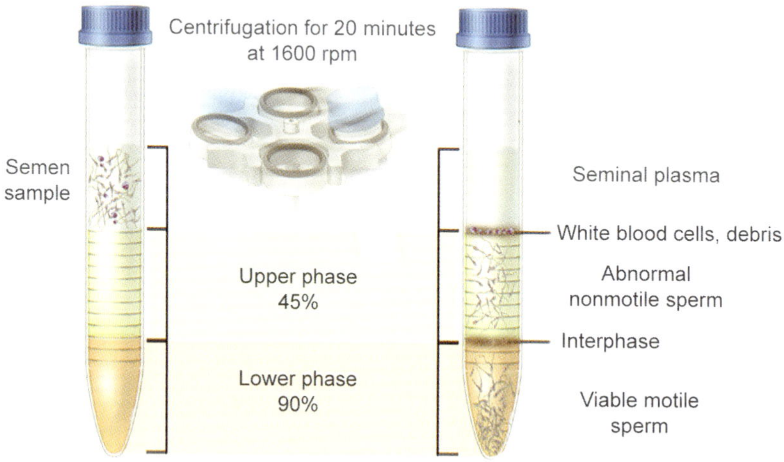

Fig. 11: Density gradient method.

Gradient media available are:

- SupraSperm (MediCult)
- IxaPrep (MediCult)
- PureSperm (Nidacon)
- Spermgrad (Shivani Scientific)
- Sil-Select (Microm, UK)

Method for SupraSperm: SupraSperm is a salt solution containing a colloidal suspension of silica particles stabilized with covalently bound hydrophilic saline.

- 2 × 1 mL of semen should be used to run two gradients for each semen sample.
- Dispense 2 mL of 55% SupraSperm to a test tube and dispense 2 mL of 80% medium underneath this with a pipette.
- Carefully dispense 1 mL of semen on top of this and centrifuge at 300 g for 20 minutes.
- Remove the supernatant and resuspend the pellet in 2–3 mL of SPM and centrifuge at 200 g for 10 minutes.
- Remove supernatant, leave pellet, and repeat the wash process.
- Finally resuspend the pellet in the desired concentration of SPM.

Final wash with culture medium to remove the gradient solution is the drawback of this method.

Variations with other media:

- *IxaPrep:* It has two pure cell separating agents—polysucrose and iodixanol with HEPES buffer. Top layer has SPM + polysucrose. Bottom layer has SPM + polysucrose + iodixanol. Semen preparation is done in the same way.
- *Scandinavian method (SpermGrad):* Bottom layer has 90% and upper layer has 45% and washing is done with G Fert.
- *PureSperm (Gradient method):* It has 90% and 45% solution. First centrifugation is 500 g for 10 minutes, and the other two centrifugations are 250 g for 5 minutes.
- *Sil-Select gradient method:* It has 80% and 40% solutions and centrifugation is done at 300–600 g for 10–20 minutes.

Gradient media are available as ready-made media where two separate media of different density are available. Media are also available as 100% media. These can be diluted to desired densities using flushing media. If, for example, 45% gradient medium is to be made, in a syringe of 1 mL, 0.45 mL of 100% gradient medium is taken and to that 0.55 mL of flushing medium is added.

If the usage is higher the preparation can also be made in samples of 10 mL.

Tips for a better yield of sperms in gradient method:

- Longer centrifugation time increases the recovery of both motile and immotile sperms.
- Higher centrifugation speed increases recovery of motile sperms and low-density particles, so shorter time is required with higher speeds.
- Because of the low density, debris, round cells and the abnormal sperms with amorphous heads, and cytoplasmic droplets never reach the bottom of the tube.

Density gradient method is generally thought to be superior to other two techniques, as it gives more morphologically normal sperms with grade A motility and normal DNA integrity with less chromatin and nuclear DNA anomalies in prepared sample. It also reduces ROS and leukocyte concentration. Though a Cochrane review of Boomsma et al. showed, in a meta-analysis, that there was no evidence of a difference in effectiveness of a swim up versus density gradient method on pregnancy rates per couple. Swim-up technique versus wash and centrifugation also showed no significant difference in pregnancy rates.[5] So, no one sperm preparation method is better than other in present scenario, though it depends on the nature of semen sample. Recovery rate of sperms after swim up is lower (<20%) as compared to that with density gradient method, which is >20%.[6]

Current paper by Vagios et al. found that overall, there is no difference in clinical pregnancy or live-birth rate between patients for whom simple wash or density gradient was used for semen preparation for IUI. So simple wash can be cost-effective and time-effective (saving).[7]

PREPARATION FROM THE FROZEN SAMPLE

- Thaw the specimen 30 minutes before IUI
- Place frozen vials in 37°C water bath for 10 minutes.
- Shake vials gently to confirm the disappearance of ice crystals.
- Then treat as a fresh sample.

Newer methods for sperm preparation like selection based on sperm surface charge and nonapoptotic sperm selection are at present used only for IVF. Selection based on sperm surface charge method is based on electrophoresis-based technology and electronegative charge on the sperm. CD52 (a specific surface protein) is correlated with normal sperm morphology and capacitation.

This technique is used in samples with high DNA damage. Zeta method selects sperms with respect to membrane surface charges or Zeta potential. This method has been found to increase fertilization, implantation, and pregnancy rates.[8]

Nonapoptotic Sperm Selection

This method utilizes magnetic cell sorting (MACS) using Annexin V MicroBeads.[8]

In Cases of Retrograde Ejaculation

Patient first empties his bladder. Then alkalizer is given to the patient. After sometime, he is asked to masturbate. The urine sample is collected in culture media and is centrifuged at 500 g for 8 minutes. The supernatant is removed and pellet is washed by gradient method.

HIV-positive Sample

Human immunodeficiency viruses are found in plasma. They are not inside the sperm cell. Here, semen is prepared by gradient method followed by swim up. Then the sample can be used for IUI.

CARRY HOME MESSAGE

- For regular IUI, swim up is a very good method and is much cheaper than density gradient method.
- We have observed that pregnancy rate is very high with 8–10 million postwash count.
- It is very vital that you select a method and modify it to achieve that count.
- We can have our own modification for speed of centrifugation and time of centrifugation according to the count and motility of the sample.

REFERENCES

1. Nijs M. Study of sperm parameters in assisted reproduction outcome. Maastricht, The Netherlands: Datawyse Bockproducties; 2009.
2. Bjorndahl L, Mortimer D, Barratt C, Castilla JA, Menkveld R, Kvist U. Practical guide to basic Laboratory Andrology. Cambridge: Cambridge University Press; 2010.
3. World Health Organization. Laboratory Annual for the Examination of Human Semen and Semen-cervical Mucus Interaction, 5th edition. New York: Cambridge University Press; 2010. p. 287.
4. Fauque P, Lehert P, Lamotte M, Bettahar-Lebugle K, Bailly A, Diligent C, et al. Clinical success of intrauterine insemination cycles is affected by the sperm preparation time. Fertil Steril. 2014;101(6):1618-23.
5. Boomsma CM, Heineman MJ, Cohlen BJ, Farquhar C. Semen preparation techniques for intrauterine insemination. Cochrane Database Syst Rev. 2007;(4):CD004507.
6. World Health Organization. WHO Laboratory Manual for Examination and Processing of Human Semen, 5th edition. Geneva: WHO Press; 2010.
7. Vagios S, Velmahos CS, Cheroveim P, Dimitriadis I, Bormann CL. The impact of different sperm preparation methos on clinical pregnancy and live birth rates in intrauterine insemination cycles: a retrospective single center cohort study. Fertil Steril. 2023;120(3):617-24.
8. Said TM, Land JA. Effects of advanced selection methods on sperm quality and ART outcome: a systematic review. Hum Reprod Update. 2011;17(6):719-33.

Index

Page numbers followed by *f* refer to figure and *t* refer to table.